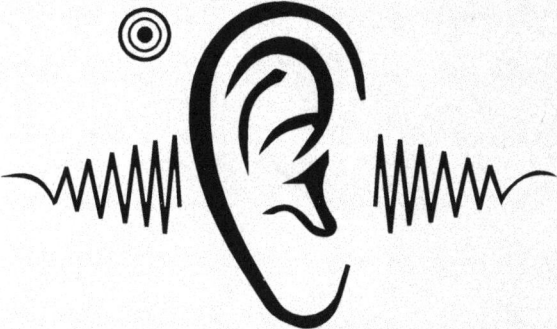

MY ACOUSTIC
NEMESIS

Russell Holden

❖ Pixel Tweaks Publications
SELF-PUBLISHING MADE SIMPLE

First published in 2016
© Pixel Tweaks

Upated 2020

ISBN: 978-1-9998936-2-0

Book interior Design by Russell Holden
Cover design inspired by Jamie Holden

www.pixeltweakspublications.com

Pixel Tweaks Publications
SELF-PUBLISHING MADE SIMPLE

Thanks to everyone who

got me to where I am today

This book is dedicated to my children
Jamie & Niamh
Max & Holly
and my granddaughters
Bonnie & Margot

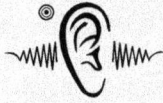

Contents

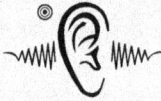

Introduction

Like most people diagnosed with an acoustic neuroma I had never heard of this condition nor what to expect post-operation or indeed how my life would change. So I did what we all do for informed medical information these days, I Googled it!

I found a wealth of information on the Acoustic Neuroma Association web site and others like it. At the time many of these sites provided medical information but I wanted true-life experiences. This was in the days before blogging had become a thing, but there were many 'diary' sites. I thought it would be good to get the worst-case scenario and view anything else as a bonus. I soon learned that a person's experience varies depending on age, size & position of the tumour removed and general health. One site that caught my eye was a US patient's Acoustic Neuroma diary website. Following his surgery, he had made a daily report of his recovery for a few months and added updates for the next couple of years. It was a great source of inspiration and encouragement to me – that there was life after acoustic neuroma. I decided to make a note of my experience to share with any about to undergo the same operation.

I have included lots of photographs of my experiences. Some of these show the aftermath of operations and include pictures of bloody dressings and scarring. I also apologise in advance for the many photos of my ugly mug!

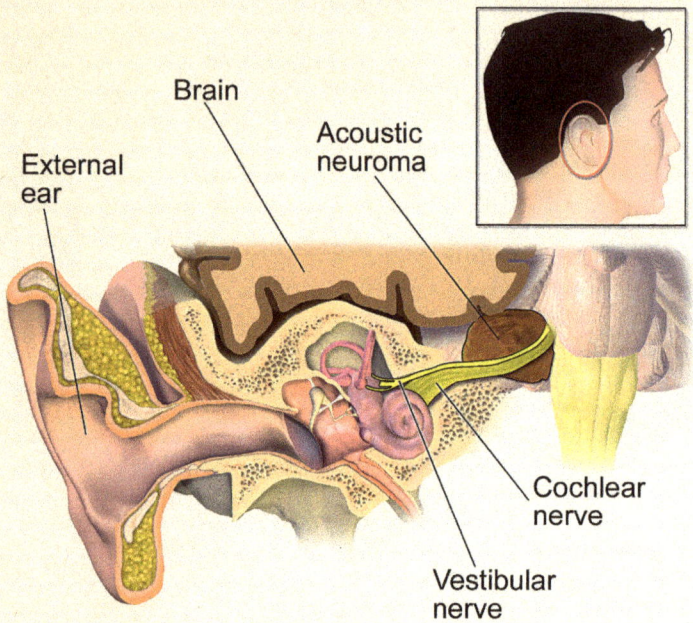

External ear

Brain

Acoustic neuroma

Cochlear nerve

Vestibular nerve

Acoustic Neuroma

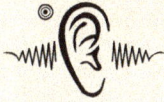

What is An Acoustic Neuroma?

This section contains an overview of information about the condition I gleaned from various resources. The references are at the end of the chapter. There's quite a bit of medical jargon so feel free to move to the next chapter!

Acoustic neuromas, the common term for vestibular schwannomas, are neither 'acoustic' nor neuromas since they do not arise from nerve tissue itself. In essence, acoustic neuromas develop from an overproduction of non-neuronal glial (Schwann) cells that support and protect the vestibular (balance) portion of the vestibulocochlear nerve. They are slow-growing local, benign and non-invasive. Progression to malignancy in this kind of tumour is rare. They usually develop gradually over a period of years, expanding at their site of origin roughly 1–2 mm each year; however, up to 50% of such tumours do not grow at all, at least for many years after diagnosis.

Tumour growth may be erratic, alternating between periods of relative dormancy or very slow growth and rapid growth. Tumours are typically described as small (less than 1.5

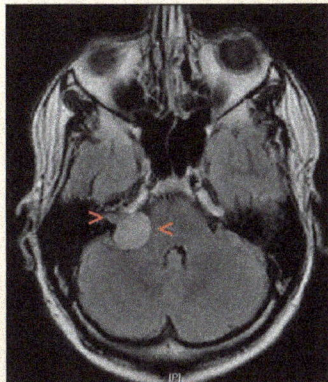

cm), medium (1.5 cm to 2.5 cm), large (2.5 cm to 4 cm), or giant (greater than 4 cm). Tumours are described by a combination of their location and size. An intracanalicular tumour is small and in the internal auditory canal. A cisternal tumour extends outside the auditory canal. A compressive tumour infringes upon the cerebellum or brainstem. Very large tumours may obstruct cerebrospinal fluid drainage.

The tumour may develop within the auditory canal, where the vestibulocochlear nerve which supplies the inner ear penetrates the skull (intracanalicular neuroma) or outside the canal (extra-canalicular neuroma). The vestibulocochlear nerve has two components, the auditory and vestibular portions. Most schwannomas start out as intracanalicular, and growth compresses the nerve against the bony canal, so the first symptoms of the tumour are unilateral sensorineural hearing loss or distubances in balance. It may also compress the labyrinthine artery (main artery supplying the vestibular apparatus and cochlea of the inner ear) which passes through the auditory canal, resulting in ischemia or infarction ('heart attack' of the ear, resulting in death of the supplied tissue).

A vestibular schwannoma is a benign primary intracranial tumour of the myelin-forming cells of the vestibulocochlear nerve (8th cranial nerve). A type of schwannoma, this tumour arises from the Schwann cells responsible for the myelin sheath that helps keep peripheral nerves insulated. The incidence is approximately 2 per 100,000 per year. That equates to 1200 new diagnoses per year assuming a UK population of 60 million. Based on MRI studies, the true prevalence may be around 0.05% (1 in 200) of the population, which equates to 30,000 people, also assuming a UK population of 60 million. Approximately 2,000 to 3,000 cases are diagnosed each year in the United States (6 to 9 per million persons). Comprehensive studies from Denmark published in 2012 showed an annual incidence of 19-23 per million from 2002 to 2008, over the last 30 years the reported incidence have been increasing, until the last decade in which an approximation of the true incidence may have been found. Most recent publications suggest that the incidence of vestibular schwannomas have been rising because of advances in MRI scanning.

Most cases are diagnosed in people between the ages of 30 and 60, and men and women appear to be affected equally. Most vestibular schwannomas occur spontaneously in those without a family history. The primary symptoms of vestibular schwannoma are unexplained progressive unilateral hearing loss and tinnitus, and vestibular (disequilibrium) symptoms. Treatment of the condition is by surgery or radiation, and often results in substantial or complete hearing loss in the affected ear. Observation (non-treatment) over time also usually results in hearing loss in the affected ear.

Signs and symptoms

Early symptoms are easily overlooked, sometimes mistaken for the normal changes of aging or attributed to noise exposure earlier in life, often delaying diagnosis. The most prevalent symptoms in patients suffering from vestibular schwannoma is hearing loss (94 %), tinnitus (83 %) and vertigo (49 %).

Hearing loss

The first symptom in 90% of those with an acoustic neuroma is unexplained unilateral sensorineural hearing loss, meaning there is damage to the inner ear (cochlea) or nerve pathways from the inner ear to the brain. It involves a reduction in sound level, speech understanding and hearing clarity. In about 70 percent of cases there is a high frequency pattern of loss. The loss of hearing is usually subtle and worsens slowly, although occasionally a sudden loss of hearing may occur(i.e. sudden deafness). Hearing loss can vary from mild hearing loss to complete deafness.

Tinnitus

Unilateral tinnitus (ringing or hissing in the ears) is also a hallmark symptom of acoustic neuroma. Not all patients with tinnitus have acoustic neuroma and not all AN patients have tinnitus. Most of them do however, both before and after treatment.

Balance

Since the balance portion of the eighth nerve is where the tumour arises, unsteadiness and balance problems or even vertigo (the feeling like the world is spinning), may occur during the growth of the tumour. The remainder of the balance system sometimes compensates for this loss, and, in some cases, no imbalance will be noticed. Balance or vertigo is the third most common symptom in patients with acoustic neuromas (50% incidence). The onset of these may be subtle, like disorientation in dark hallways, and be dismissed as age related decline. These symptoms tend to occur later in the development of the tumour.

Pressure in the ear

Vestibular schwannoma patients sometimes complain of a feeling that their ear is plugged or "full".

Facial weakness or paralysis

Larger tumours can press on the trigeminal nerve (CN V), causing facial numbness and tingling - constantly or intermittently. The facial nerve (CN VII) is rarely affected in the same way; however, due to its proximity to some structures of the inner and middle ear, it can be damaged during radiological treatment or surgical removal of the tumour, particularly in the case of large growths.

At the time some people learn they have an acoustic neuroma, they are also told that this tumour may involve the nerve that controls facial movement. However, it is much more common for treatment, rather than the tumour itself, to damage this nerve, leading to weakness or paralysis of the face. Taste, a sensation that reflects accurately sweet, sour, bitter and bland, is also a function of the facial nerve. Should any of the cranial nerves be damaged or need to be cut during surgery, it is sometimes possible for a neurosurgeon to microsuture the ends together; however, this is a new and very delicate specialist procedure, where long recovery times, incomplete healing and some permanent loss of function are to be expected.

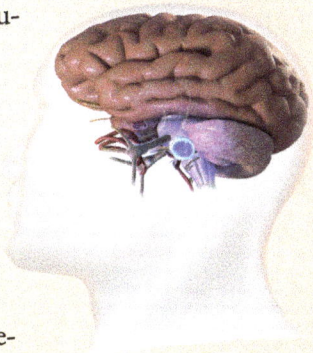

Headache

Recurring headaches are an uncommon symptom, also tending to occur only in cases of larger tumours.

Advanced symptoms

Large tumours may cause disabling and life-threatening symptoms. Large tumours that compress the adjacent brainstem may affect other local cranial nerves. The glossopharyngeal and vagus nerves are uncommonly involved, but their involvement may lead to altered gag or swallowing reflexes.

Larger tumours may lead to increased intracranial pressure, with its associated symptoms such as headache, vomiting, clumsy gait and mental confusion. This can be a life-threatening complication requiring urgent treatment.

Cause

The cause of acoustic neuromas is usually unknown; however there is a growing body of evidence that sporadic defects in tumour suppressor genes may give rise to these tumours in some individuals. In particular, loss or mutation of a tumour suppressor gene on the long arm of chromosome 22 is strongly associated with vestibular schwannomas.Other studies have hinted at exposure to loud noise on a consistent basis. One study has shown a relationship between acoustic neuromas and prior exposure to head and neck radiation, and a concomitant history of having had a parathyroid adenoma (tumour found in proximity to the thyroid gland controlling calcium metabolism). There are even controversies on hand held cellular phones. Whether or not the radiofrequency radiation has anything to do with acoustic neuroma formation, remains to be seen. To date, no environmental factor (such as cell phones or diet) has been scientifically proven to cause these tumours. The Acoustic Neuroma Association (ANA) does recommend that frequent cellular phone users use a hands free device to enable separation of the device from the head.

Although there is an inheritable condition called Neurofibromatosis Type 2 (NF2) which can lead to acoustic neuroma formation in some people, most acoustic neuromas occur spontaneously without any evidence of family history (95%). NF2 occurs with a frequency of 1 in 30,000 to 1 in 50,000 births. The hallmark of this disorder is bilateral acoustic neuromas (an acoustic neuroma on both sides) usually developing in late childhood or early adulthood, frequently associated with other brain and spinal chord tumours.

Pathophysiology

As intracanalicular tumours grow, they tend to expand into the cerebellopontine angle (CPA), leading to their characteristic "ice-cream-cone like" appearance on a radiograph. When the tumour expands extracanalicularly, the growth rate often increases, since it is no longer confined by the bony auditory canal. As the schwannoma expands into the CPA, it may infringe on cranial nerve V (controls facial sensation, chewing and swallowing) and cranial nerve VII (controls facial expression and taste). Cranial nerve VIII, along with these two nerves, also passes through the CPA, so more serious or complete hearing loss and episodes of vertigo may occur as the tumour infringes on it there.

When a schwannoma becomes large, it can displace normal brain tissue. The brain is not invaded by the tumour, but the tumour pushes the brain as it enlarges. Vital functions to sustain life can be threatened when large tumours cause severe pressure on the brainstem and cerebellum.

Very large tumours may compress or distort the spinal fluid spaces, resulting in hydrocephalus, with symptoms of headaches, vomiting, nausea, sleepiness and eventually coma.

Diagnosis

The Gold Standard for diagnosis of vestibular schwannoma is without doubt Gadolinium enhanced magnetic resonance imaging (MRI) yet several examinations may arise suspicion of vestibular schwannomas.

Routine auditory tests may reveal a loss of hearing and speech discrimination (the patient may hear sounds in that ear, but cannot comprehend what is being said). Pure tone audiometry should be performed to effectively evaluate hearing in both ears. In some clinics the clinical criteria for follow up testing for AN is a 15 dB differential in thresholds between ears for three consecutive frequencies.

An auditory brainstem response test is a much more cost effective screening alternative to MRI for those at low risk of AN. This test provides information on the passage of an electrical impulse along the circuit from the inner ear to the brainstem pathways. An acoustic neuroma can interfere with the passage of this electrical impulse through the hearing nerve at the site of tumour growth in the internal auditory canal, even when hearing is still essentially normal. This implies the possible diagnosis of an acoustic neuroma when the test result is abnormal. An abnormal auditory brainstem response test should be followed by an MRI. The sensitivity of this test is proportional to the tumour size - the smaller the tumour, the more likely is a false negative result; small tumours within the auditory canal will often be missed. However, since these tumours would usually be watched rather than treated, the clinical significance of overlooking them may be negligible.

Advances in scanning and testing have made possible the identification of small acoustic neuromas (those still confined to the internal auditory canal). MRI using Gadolinium as an enhancing contrast material is the preferred diagnostic test for identifying acoustic neuromas. The image formed clearly defines an acoustic neuroma if it is present and this technique can identify tumours measuring down to 5 millimeters in diameter (the scan spacing).

When an MRI is not available or cannot be performed, a computerized tomography scan (CT scan) with contrast is suggested for patients in whom an acoustic neuroma is suspected. The combination of CT scan and audiogram approach the reliability of MRI in making the diagnosis of acoustic neuroma.

Treatment

There are three treatment options available to a patient. These options are observation, microsurgical removal and radiation (radiosurgery or radiotherapy). Determining which treatment to choose involves consideration of many factors including the size of the tumour, its location, the patient's age, physical health and current symptoms. About 25% of all acoustic neuromas are treated with medical management consisting of a periodic monitoring of the patient's neurological status, serial imaging studies, and the use of hearing aids when appropriate. One of the last great obstacles in the management of acoustic neuromas is hearing preservation and/or rehabilitation after hearing loss. Hearing loss is both a symptom and concommitant risk, regardless of the treatment option chosen. Treatment does not restore hearing already lost, though there are a few rare cases of hearing recovery reported.

A diagnosis of NF2 related bilateral acoustic neuromas creates the possibility of complete deafness if the tumours are left to grow unchecked. Preventing or treating the complete deafness that may befall individuals with NF2 requires complex decision making. The trend at most medical centres is to recommend treatment for the smallest tumour which has the best chance of preserving hearing. If this goal is successful, then treatment can also be offered for the remaining tumour. If hearing is not preserved at the initial treatment, then usually the second tumour, in the only-hearing ear, is just observed. If it shows continued growth and becomes life-threatening, or if the hearing is lost over time as the tumour grows, then treatment is undertaken. This strategy has the highest chance of preserving hearing for the longest time possible.

Observation

Since acoustic neuromas tend to be slow-growing and are benign tumours, careful observation over a period of time may be appropriate for some patients. When a small tumour is discovered in an older patient, observation to determine the growth rate of the tumour may be indicated if serious symptoms are not present. There is now good evidence from large observational studies that suggest many small tumours in older individuals do not grow, thus allowing tumours with no growth to be observed successfully. If the tumour grows, treatment may become necessary. Another example of a group of patients for whom observation may be indicated includes patients with a tumour in their only hearing or better hearing ear, particularly when the tumour is of a size that hearing preservation with treatment would be unlikely. In this group of patients, MRI is used to follow the growth pattern. Treatment is recommended if either the hearing is lost or the tumour size becomes life-threatening, thus allowing the patient to retain hearing for as long as possible.

Current studies suggest surgeons should observe small acoustic neuromas (those 1.5 cm or less). Over a period of 10 years of observation with no treatment, 45% of patients with small tumours (and therefore minimal symptoms) lose functional hearing on the affected side; this percentage is considerably higher than that for patients actively treated with hearing-preserving microsurgery or radiosurgery.

Surgery

The goals of surgery are to control the tumour, and preserve function of the involved nerves (i.e. those involved in facial musculature and hearing). Preservation of hearing is an important goal for patients who present with functional hearing. Surgery cannot restore hearing already lost.

Microsurgical tumour removal can be done at one of three levels: subtotal removal, near total removal or total tumour removal. Many tumours can be entirely removed by surgery. Microsurgical techniques and instruments, along with the operating microscope, have greatly reduced the surgical risks of total tumour removal. Subtotal removal is indicated when anything further risks life or neurological function. In these cases the residual tumour should be followed for risk of growth (approximately 35%). If the residual grows further, treatment will likely be required. Periodic MRI studies are important to follow the potential growth rate of any tumour. Near total tumour removal is used when small areas of the tumour are so adherent to the facial nerve that total removal would result in facial weakness. The piece left is generally less than 1% of the original and poses a risk of regrowth of approximately 3%.

There are three main surgical approaches for the removal of an acoustic neuroma: **translabyrinthine, retrosigmoid/ sub-occipital and middle fossa.** The approach used for each individual person is based on several factors such as tumour size, location, skill and experience of the surgeon, and whether hearing preservation is a goal. Each of the surgical approaches has advantages and disadvantages in terms of ease of tumour removal, likelihood of preservation of facial nerve function and hearing, and post-operative complications.

During surgery, intraoperative neurophysiological monitoring of the facial, acoustic and lower cranial nerves can reduce the risk of injury. In particular, following the 1991 NIH National institutes of Health Acoustic Neuroma Consensus Panel, the use of facial nerve monitoring has become a standard practice in the United States to reduce the risk of facial paralysis. With massive tumours that compress the brainstem and cerebellum, staged surgical approaches or subtotal surgical resection followed by stereotactic radiosurgery may reduce the risks to life, brain and cranial nerves.

Translabyrinthine approach

The translabyrinthine approach may be preferred by the surgical team when the patient has no useful hearing, or when an attempt to preserve hearing would be impractical. The incision for this approach is located behind the ear and allows excellent exposure of the internal auditory canal and tumour. Since the incision goes directly through the inner ear, this results in permanent and complete hearing loss in that ear. Many patients with medium to large ANs have no functional hearing in the ear anyway, so this may not be an issue. The surgeon has the advantage of knowing the location of the facial nerve prior to tumour dissection and removal. Any size tumour can be removed with this approach and this approach affords the least likelihood of long-term postoperative headaches.

Retrosigmoid/sub-occipital approach

The incision for this approach is located in a slightly different location. This approach creates an opening in the skull behind the mastoid part of the ear, near the back of the head on the side of the tumour. The surgeon exposes the tumour from its posterior (back) surface, thereby getting a very good view of the tumour in relation to the brainstem. When removing large tumours through this approach, the facial nerve can be exposed by early opening of the internal auditory canal. Any size tumour can be removed with this approach. One of the main advantages of the retrosigmoid approach is the possibility of preserving hearing. For small tumours, a disadvantage lies in the risk of long-term postoperative headache.

Middle fossa approach

This approach is in a slightly different incision location and is utilized primarily for the purpose of hearing preservation in patients with small tumours, typically confined to the internal auditory canal. A small window of bone is removed above the ear canal to allow exposure of the tumour from the upper surface of the internal auditory canal, preserving the inner ear structures.

Cancers (radiotherapy)

There are documented incidences of new malignant gliomas and malignant progression of ANs after focused radiotherapy using either SRS or FRT for benign intracranial lesions.

Tinnitus

Most patients present with tinnitus before treatment, and also have it after treatment. About one in 5 patients without tinnitus acquire it, and for about 2 in 5 with tinnitus it resolves or decreases.

Hearing loss

While formerly, preservation of hearing during treatment was very unlikely, the newer techniques of microsurgery and stereotactic radiotherapy have enabled the preservation of functional hearing in the majority of cases. Overall, 60-66% of persons treated for acoustic neuroma preserve their hearing. Likelihood of preserving hearing is correlated with better hearing pre-treatment, and smaller size of tumour. Even in those with functional hearing following surgery or radiotherapy, hearing may decline for years afterward.

Tumour re-growth

Tumour regrowth occurs in 1-3% of cases treated surgically, and 14% in cases treated with radiation. Likelihood of regrowth is proportional to the bulk of tumour remaining in case of surgery, and inversely proportional to radiation dose in case of radiotherapy. In case retreatment with surgery following radiation was required, the rate of complications was from 19.4% to 27% in two different studies, because the tumour tends to fuse to the nerve.

Facial nerve damage

In the 2012 Acoustic Neuroma Association patient survey, 29% of the respondents reported facial weakness or paralysis, some of which were pre- and some were post-treatment. This represents a significant improvement from the 1998 Acoustic Neuroma Association patient survey of post-treatment acoustic neuroma patients, which revealed that at the time they completed the survey, only 59% were satisfied with the appearance of their face. Treatment for an acoustic neuroma may damage the facial nerve – either with surgery or radiation. It is usually possible, however, to preserve some degree of facial function even in cases where the nerve is extensively involved. For those with partial nerve regeneration, in whom some facial weakness remains, non-surgical facial rehabilitation therapies also may be beneficial.

Taste disturbance and mouth dryness

Taste disturbance and mouth dryness are frequent for a few weeks following surgery. In a few patients this disturbance is longer or permanent.

Headaches

Head pain is expected in most patients immediately after acoustic neuroma surgery (acute phase) because of the incision, variations in cerebrospinal fluid pressure, muscle pain, or even meningitic pain. It typically responds to appropriate medications and resolves within several weeks. Headache that persists for months or even years after surgery (chronic phase) can be debilitating and may be an under-appreciated complication of acoustic neuroma treatment. In patients who experience chronic headaches, the pain often persists for prolonged periods of time, and does not always respond well to various medical and surgical treatments. The exact prevalence and causes of chronic postoperative headache (POH) are elusive. After surgical treatment of acoustic neuroma, the reported incidence of headache in the 2012 Acoustic Neuroma Association patient survey has ranged from 0% to 35% depending on the type of surgical approach, technique used and reporting interval since surgery. Frequent and severe post-operative headaches have been more often associated with the sub-occipital/retro-sigmoid approach than the translabyrinthine or middle fossa approaches.

Balance

Essentially everyone who has been treated for an acoustic neuroma experiences difficulty with balance and/or dizziness to some degree. For some, this instability may be mild and noticeable only in certain circumstances, such as ambulating with head movements, or walking in the dark. For others, there may be difficulty returning to work, or even performing regular daily activities such as driving, shopping, house work and even working on a computer.

Paralysis and death

In rare cases where large tumours infringe on the brainstem which controls motor nerves, with or without surgery, paralysis or death can result. This occurs in less than 1% of large tumours.

Radiation

Another treatment option for an acoustic neuroma is radiation. Stereotactic radiation can be delivered as single fraction stereotactic radiosurgery or as multi-session fractionated stereotactic radiotherapy. Both techniques are performed in the outpatient setting, not requiring general anesthesia or a hospital stay. The purpose of these techniques is to arrest the growth of the tumour. This treatment has not been well studied and thus it is unclear if it is better than observation or surgery.

All types of radiation therapy for acoustic neuromas may result in "tumour control" in which the tumour cells die and necrosis occurs. Tumour control means that the tumour growth may slow or stop and, in some cases, the tumour may shrink in size. Acoustic neuroma tumours have been completely eliminated by radiation treatments in almost no cases. In other words, radiation cannot remove the tumour like microsurgery would. Tumours under 2.5 - 3.0 cm, without significant involvement of the brainstem, are more favorable for radiation treatment. Side effects can occur when the brainstem is irradiated and in some cases of large tumours, radiation is suggested against.

In single dose treatments, hundreds of small beams of radiation are aimed at the tumour. This results in a concentrated dose of radiation to the tumour and avoids exposure of surrounding brain tissues to the radiation. Many patients have been successfully treated this way. Facial weakness or numbness, in the hands of experienced radiation physicians, occurs in only a small percent of cases. Hearing can be preserved in some cases.

The multi-dose treatment, FSR, delivers smaller doses of radiation over a period of time, requiring the patient to return to the treatment location on a daily basis, from 3 to 30 times, generally over several weeks. Each visit lasts a few minutes and most patients are free to go about their daily business before and after each treatment session. Early data indicates that FSR may result in better hearing preservation when compared to single-session SRS.

Radiated patients require lifetime follow-up with MRI scans. Follow-up after SRS and FSR typically involves an MRI scan and audiogram at six months, one year, then yearly for several years, then every second or third year indefinitely to make sure the tumour does not start to grow again. Patients should understand there have been rare reports of malignant degeneration (a benign tumour becoming malignant) after radiotherapy. In some cases the tumour does not die and continues to grow. In those instances, another treatment is necessary - either microsurgery or sometimes another dose of radiation.

Studies are beginning to appear for the other modalities. All of the techniques use computers to create three dimensional models of the tumour and surrounding neural structures. Radiation physicists then create dosimetry maps showing the level of radiation to be received by the tumour and the normal tissues. Surgeons, radiation therapists and physicists then modify the dosimetry to maximize tumour doses and minimize radiation toxicity to surrounding normal tissues. Treatments generally last 30–60 minutes. Just like for surgery, the experience of the team in treating acoustic neuromas with all modalities (surgery and radiation) can affect outcomes. There are a multitude of studies supporting short-term (<5 yrs.) and longer-term (over 10 yrs.) tumour control with radiation. Unfortunately, as is the case with microsurgical studies, most have inconsistent follow-up to draw definitive conclusions.

Epidemiology

Vestibular schwannoma is a rare condition: incident rate in the U.S. in 2010 was 11/1,000,000 persons, mean age 53. Occurrence was equally distributed versus age, gender and laterality. In patients with unilateral hearing loss, only about 1 in 1000 has acoustic neuroma.

American actor, director, humanitarian, social activist and film producer Mark Ruffalo (aka The Hulk) was diagnosed with vestibular schwannoma in 2001 which resulted in a period of partial facial paralysis. He recovered from the paralysis; however, he became deaf in his left ear as a result of the tumour.

REFERENCES

Acoustic Neuroma Basic Overview. Acoustic Neuroma Association. March 2015.

Hearing Loss Rehabilitation For Acoustic Neuroma Patients. Acoustic Neuroma Association. January 2013.

Facial Nerve & Acoustic Neuroma: Possible Damage & Rehabilitation. Acoustic Neuroma Association. July 2015.

Headache Associated with Acoustic Neuroma Treatment. Acoustic Neuroma Association. November 2013.

Improving Balance Associated with Acoustic Neuroma. Acoustic Neuroma Association. September 2013.

Idleman & Associates (2012). 2012 ANA Patient Survey. Acoustic Neuroma Association.

Idleman & Associates (2014). 2014 Report on ANA Patient Database. Acoustic Neuroma Association.

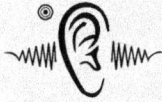

In the Beginning

My history with Acoustic Neuroma began around 1997. That was the year I first noticed a slight twinge as I rubbed my face dry one evening with the towel. It felt as if I had briefly touched a raw nerve. It was so fleeting that I didn't think much of it, however as time progressed this momentary pain grew more and more intense – sometimes when I touched my face, other times a yawn and even a gust of the wind would set off a series of facial spasms which were so excruciatingly painful I had to immediately stop whatever I was doing and let the contraction run its course. After the pain had passed, I would be left feeling punch drunk and watery-eyed.

Each year these spasms would occur more regularly and become more and more intense. They went from happening very occasionally at first to once a month, then a couple of times a month, and so on. The pain was never in the same place every-time – the spasms would 'migrate' up & down my face.

I first mentioned it to the doctor around 1999. I was given an examination and sent for a CRT scan, but nothing noticeable was found that could be causing the pain. I have never been a regular visitor to the doctors and could count on one hand the number of visits I'd had in the previous decade. I'd keep putting off visits about my spasms as I'd usually spend hours in a waiting room to see a doctor who was seemingly baffled by my ailment. After a few visits, the doctor diagnosed Trigeminal Neuralgia. It was suggested that one of the trigeminal nerves in my face had a blood vessel sitting on it which was causing the terrible facial pain.

Thus an appointment was made for a visit to the Pain Clinic at the local hospital, and I was prescribed various drugs, including Amitriptyline to control the pain. These drugs were pretty useless – they succeeded in making me feel in a constant state of lethargy but did nothing to kill the pain, and because I didn't know when one of the spasm attacks would be, I couldn't take anything to pre-empt the pain either.

One night in 2003, my daughter was feeling unwell, so slept in our bed, and I stayed in her room. There was a small clock in there, and I began to notice that I could only hear it ticking when I had my right ear on the pillow. When I turned over, I couldn't hear the ticking at all. It was the first time I realised I was losing my hearing!

On the next visit to the doctor, I mentioned that the hearing was reduced in my right ear and asked her to look for a wax blockage – she couldn't see anything at that time so sent me to the hospital for a hearing test.

The hospital confirmed there was a hearing issue but couldn't see anything with a cursory examination, so an appointment

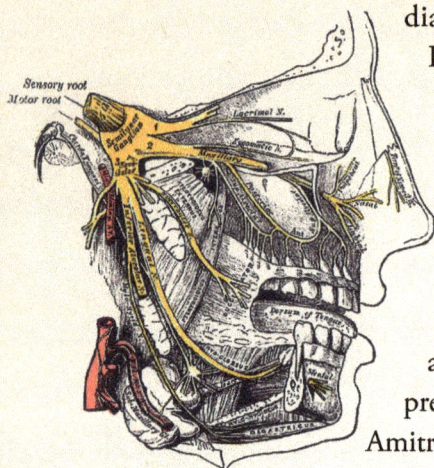

was made for me to have a more definitive MRI (Magnetic Resonance Imaging) scan.

Some weeks passed before the appointment to visit the MRI Scanner Unit popped through the letterbox. It was at my local hospital in Barrow-in-Furness, in the North West of England. At that time, they didn't have an MRI scanner installed at the hospital so a mobile unit would visit regularly.

So in January 2004, I found myself lying perfectly still in a big tube on the back of a trailer being scanned by a giant magnet!

I got the letter for an appointment for the result just a few days later (you know it's not good news when you get a reply that quick!!!)

On the day of the appointment, I went to the ENT dept and was soon called in to see the specialist Mr Stoney. Without too much preamble he told me the news.

"We found a tumour on your hearing nerve Mr Holden".

My first thought was 'at last; they have found the cause of my terrible facial pain' – it wasn't Trigeminal Neuralgia after all.

I'd never heard of an Acoustic Neuroma before – the explanation given by Mr Stoney was that it is a non-cancerous (benign) brain tumour. Also known as a vestibular schwannoma. It grows slowly over many years and doesn't tend to spread to other parts of the body.

Acoustic Neuromas grow on the nerve used for hearing and balance, which can cause problems such as hearing loss and unsteadiness.

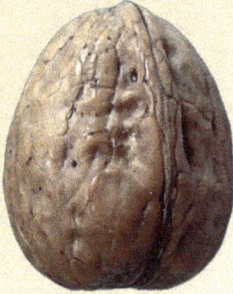

**Walnut
(actual size)**

They can sometimes be dangerous if they become too large, but most are diagnosed and treated before they reach this stage. My Acoustic Neuroma was currently approx 3cm ... the same size as a walnut!

I got an appointment to see the consultant in Manchester a fortnight later. He explained that as the tumour was touching my brain stem, the options I had were limited, and I would have to have it removed as soon as possible.

On the 1st March 2004, I was told to expect an appointment for surgery within the next three months.

We had a pre-booked holiday in the South of France planned in April so I hoped it would come after that.

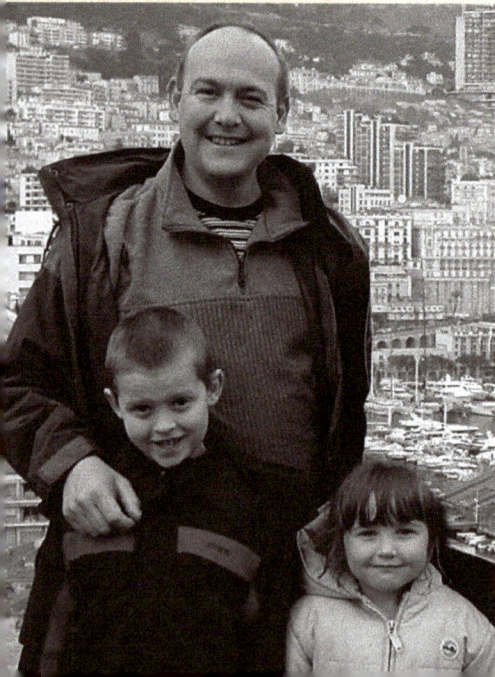

The appointment was already on my doormat the day I arrived home from France, and precisely one month after this photo was taken on a day trip to Monaco I was admitted to the Head & Neck Surgical Unit at Manchester Royal Infirmary.

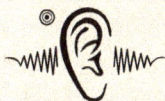

The Diary

This is a personal account of the procedure and my post operative experiences. It is not necessarily typical, and individual experiences may differ from this, but it helps to know what to expect on a daily basis.

Monday 10th May 2004

The 'invitation' to Manchester Royal Infirmary arrived sooner than I had expected and I was given just two weeks notice, so the build-up to this day wasn't too bad as I didn't have long to dwell on it.

Nicola, my wife, and I have decided to travel alone to Manchester. We said our goodbyes to the children, Jamie (age 10) and Niamh (age 5), this evening. The hospital in Manchester is 100 miles from our home, so the children are staying with their grandparents – they are to join her at the end of the week after the initial trauma of the first day's post-operation has passed. We arrived in Blackburn at my parent's home late evening, and it's from here that my mother will take us the rest of the journey to the hospital, which is then only 35 miles away. Would this be the last night I would be able to sleep on my right ear for a while?

Tuesday 11ᵗʰ May 2004

Before setting off, I had been told to phone the ward to make sure there was still a bed available for me today. As I am going into a head & neck surgical unit, there is always a chance there had been an emergency, and I might have had the operation delayed. But all was well, and I was told to come straight up to the ward on arrival.

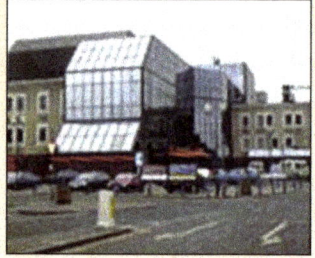

Manchester Royal Infirmary in 2004

We arrived after an uneventful journey, although finding Manchester Royal Infirmary is easier said than done. The hospital, compared to our local one in rural Cumbria, is vast! It is like a self-contained town. Very busy with lots of people coming and going.

On our arrival to the ward, I was given a bed and waited for my medical notes to arrive then I could be admitted. I was to wait four hours until 3pm for this – Nicola & my mother stayed with me to keep me company. I was experiencing lots of facial pain during most of this time, so I wasn't exactly a bundle of laughs to be with.

My Mother left us shortly afterwards but on her way out enquired at what time the following day the operation would be. We were surprised to learn the operation was to be 8:30am ON THURSDAY, the day after tomorrow! I needed an ECG and blood tests before the surgery, so I had to sit it out for a further 36 hours before the op! That evening Nicola left to stay with friends in Manchester, and I settled in for my first night as a guest of Manchester Royal Infirmary.

Wednesday 12th May 2004

After a reasonable night's sleep, I spent the morning reading, and apart from a blood test had to have no other investigation that day. Nicola arrived at 11am so we went out for the day. This was bizarre – I had imagined for weeks that I would spend this day in an operating theatre, yet here I was walking around a museum in the centre of Manchester. We had our lunch out, and I had a delicious omelette (which was to be my last full meal for a few days). We even went to the cinema! We saw a brand new Jim Carrey movie – Eternal sunshine of the spotless mind – about a man who undergoes a procedure to have his memories of a failed relationship erased. A film that takes some thinking about – not the sort to watch a few hours before going under general anaesthetic.

We returned to the ward to find it in a flurry of excitement ... we had just missed the visit of Alex Ferguson, the legendary manager of Manchester United who was visiting a family member who was on a side ward.

On returning to my bed, a member of the surgical team came to visit & explained the procedure in detail.

Under general anaesthetic, an incision is to be cut in the shape of a big 'C' around the ear. This is then peeled back, and a hole will be drilled into the skull. The tumour is then removed with the aid of a microscope little by little, to prevent too much damage to the nerves. This hole is then plugged with a skin graft taken from my stomach, and I will have a drain inserted into my spine to remove any excess fluid caused by the procedure.

Sounded delightful – I'm glad I'll be asleep! I did ask what the mortality rate is for this operation. Prof. Ramsden who was to perform the procedure was very experienced, and he had performed acoustic neuroma removal surgery thousands of times with an almost 100% success rate – I liked those odds, so it made me feel a lot more positive about the operation.

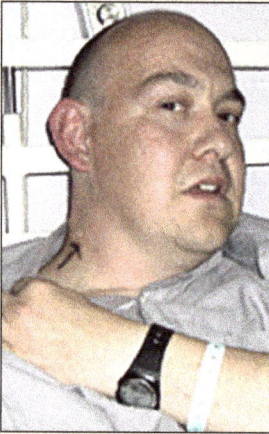

Before he left, he took out a marker pen and drew an arrow on my neck to remind the surgeon which side to cut open.

That evening I said my goodbyes to Nicola & my Mother; quite an emotional time not knowing what to feel, and without being too melodramatic this could be the last time we see each other.

Thursday 13th May (OPERATION DATE)

I was awake by 7am, after a surprisingly restful sleep – I am ready for this operation now, I have had enough of the excruciating facial pain that has dominated my life for so long. I have come to terms with the consequences of the operation, the deafness, the balance issues, the painful recovery, and now I want to get on with it and start the rest of my life.

I spent the day trying to keep my mind off the actual operation that was looming. After dinner (which I obviously couldn't partake of) I had a shower, donned my gown & DVT stockings (very fetching elasticated stockings to minimise the risk of deep vein thrombosis developing while being in a stationary position for many hours) and sat patiently waiting for the porter to take me to the last place I would hear in stereo.

I was taken to the operating theatre at 8.30pm. The anaesthetist prepared a cannula in my left hand and then attempted to put a drain into my spine. Very unpleasant, just the thought of this now makes we wince. A local anaesthetic was put in my lower spine, but they had difficulty injecting the needle in the right spot for the tap and gave up after THREE ATTEMPTS!

"Never mind," said the anaesthetist "we'll do it post-op instead". (I was to suffer back pain in that vicinity for years to come ... then in 2014 I had the experience of another three failed attempts when being tested for meningitis).

At this point, the general anaesthetic was administered. I remember lying down ... and nothing more. Whenever I have had anaesthetic in the past, I always recall the moment they say

"Count back from 10." But this time ... nothing.

I awoke to a voice that seemed to be in the distance saying,

"Russell, the operation is over with, you are in the High Dependency ward."

It was 7.30pm I had been in theatre under general anaesthetic for TEN HOURS. I fell in and out of consciousness. The next thing I remember is Nicola & my Mother coming in to see me looking very relieved that I had made it. I felt very tired.

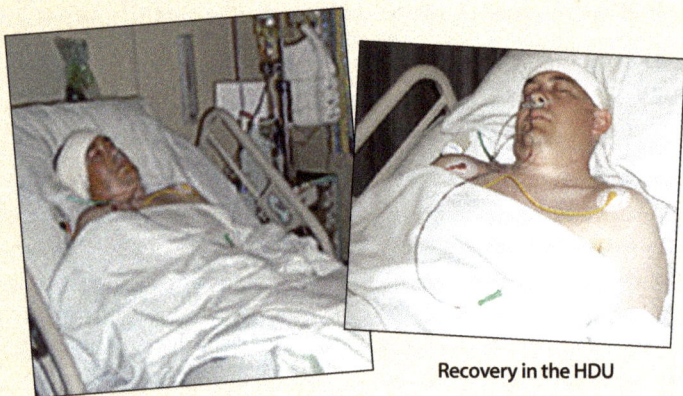

Recovery in the HDU

Friday 14th May (1 DAY POST OP)

I remember vomiting water. I felt very nauseous and had a terrific headache. My head was bandaged up, and I was on a morphine drip which I could control with a push-button. At one point, I lost my grip of the button and couldn't move my head to see where it was to pick it up again.

The consultant came to see me this morning with the news that he had managed to remove the entire tumour. He also

Apologies for the low quality of some of the photos - only the low res website versions remain told me my facial nerve had been cut but wasn't too severely damaged however it would take some time for my facial movements to return (although I could never expect the same animation on the right side of my face as I had before).

Saturday 15th May (2 DAYS POST OP)

I had a terribly disturbed night and spent much of it worrying that my lumbar drain would come out and have to go through the bother of having it put in again. I am very uncomfortable. I have a cannula in my hand, a catheter in my bladder, a tube in my spine, oxygen spectacles up my nose and a big bandage on my head – I feel the need to be free!

It is during today that I begin to feel my face drooping. The right side is now almost paralysed, I can just about close my eyelid, but not all the way, so this is causing discomfort. I was given drops to lubricate my eyeballs, so that helps a little.

My appetite is slowly returning; I had small portions of the meals served today. The children came to visit this afternoon – a welcome sight. My son was a little subdued at seeing me, but my daughter chatted away as if nothing had happened. They were both interested to see my catheter and found my newfound lack of facial expression very amusing, and imitated my lop-sided smiles. The nurse taped my eyelid down with surgical tape tonight to prevent damage which helped a great deal.

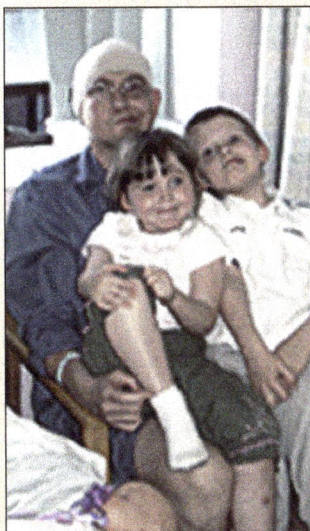

A visit from Jamie & Niamh

Sunday 16th May (3 DAYS POST OP)

I am now in a full hospital routine; each day, I awake at 4am and wait for dawn. I drift back to sleep until around 6am then lie there waiting for the day to begin. At 7.30am the nurses come round with morning medicine, and the breakfast wagon comes shortly afterwards. The doctors make their rounds at 8am, and a cup of tea is served soon after. Then just another five hours to kill before visiting time!

By Sunday I have lost another couple of tubes – the cannula has been unhooked from my hand, and I don't need the oxygen specs any more. I am feeling a lot better, although I am still in general discomfort. I get headaches but not as bad as I thought. There is a ready supply of paracetamol for the pain when it comes. By today I was being urged to go to the toilet to move my bowels. Apparently, constipation could prove damaging to the cerebral cortex, which is weakened after an Acoustic Neuroma removal, so everyone is keen to see you go. But, when you are confined to a bed with tubes attached, it isn't straightforward to go anywhere. It had been three days since my last bowel movement, and I've had laxatives poured down me since then, but the thought of sitting on a commode was the last thing I needed to encourage me to go.

I experienced severe headaches again tonight – not constant, they come in ever-intensifying waves then subside.

My right eye is a cause of significant discomfort, and I can't close my eyelid to keep it lubricated, so it keeps drying out. The windows are open on the ward, and there is a fan on which makes my eye worse. I have blurred and double vision as a result of this so I can't even read properly. I take to wearing sunglasses to protect my eyes from the breezes.

Monday 17th May
(4 DAYS POST OP)

A very special moment occurred at midnight today – the catheter came out! Not the most delightful experience in the world, but at least it was quick. The nurse 'kindly' showed me how it worked afterwards and pointed out the balloon, which is inflated in the bladder – too much information. By 9am my spinal drain was also removed – utterly free at last from tubes and more tubes, although I still can't stand by myself let alone get out of bed.

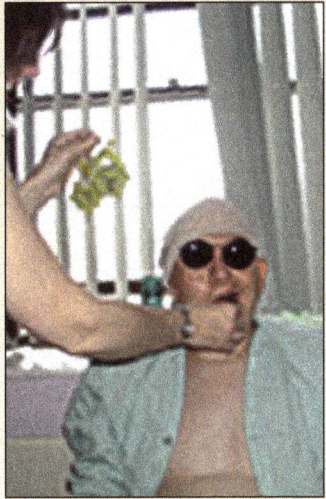

Feeding time - note the glasses to protect my 'all-seeing' eye

The nurses as ever are great, they care for your every need but don't mollycoddle - they want the patient up and about as soon as possible - they need the beds! So very soon they had me up and about and before the end of the day I was walking, with assistance, to the bathroom and yes, by 6.30pm the eagle had landed, I finally got rid of that blooming omelette, and I could breathe a sigh of relief that the laxatives were working at last.

Tuesday 18th May (5 DAYS POST OP)

Today I was put back into a traditional hospital bed, unlike the motorised one I had been in thus far. Not as high tech but more comfortable and I managed a half-decent sleep. I can now walk unaided back and forth and have been told that I will be able to go home on Thursday if this progress is maintained. I am even able to accompany visitors down the ward when they are leaving. The walking technique I have adopted is much like a tightrope walker's stance - one tentative foot at a time standing straight up with eyes looking straight ahead. I feel ready to go home now.

Wednesday 19th May (6 DAYS POST OP)

I have *another* restless night, the vivid dreams are still bugging me, it must me the brain trying to make sense of all that has happened. The headaches are less frequent and can be controlled with paracetamol. Codeine is also offered but they give you constipation and we don't want that do we? My parents came to visit this evening and I was able to walk out of the ward and down to the cafeteria with them. Each day I continue to get a little bit of my strength back.

Thursday 20th May (7 DAYS POST OP)

The doctors came round at 8am as usual and gave me the all-clear – finally, I could go home. A nurse took the staples out of my side where the skin graft was taken and from my head. This was an unusual experience – not painful but slightly uncomfortable, she snipped the staple in the middle and dragged either end out. I was fine until she ran off to get some tissue quickly as one of the holes had started to bleed, and then I felt it drip down my neck. Yuck!

I put on my 'civilian' clothes at midday – It felt soooo good to be out of the DVT stockings at last. My good friend Grahame had offered to give me a ride back home to Cumbria and arrived shortly after 1pm. We had to wait a further two hours for the prescription drugs I had to take home with me (this consisted of paracetamol, codeine, laxative and indigestion tablets).

At last, the moment arrived to leave, and it was a strange feeling walking out of the hospital after such an extended stay. It is approx 100 miles from Manchester to my home in Cumbria, so I prepared for the journey with some anti-sickness pills.

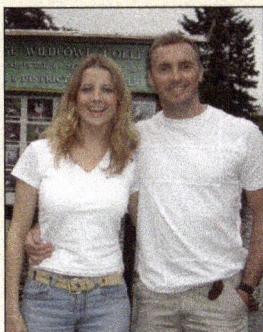

My good friend Grahame and his wife Jolene.

The trip was uneventful; we stopped on the way for a coffee and a snack – everything tastes so rich at the moment. I had a chocolate biscuit, but it felt like I'd eaten an entire gateau!

We arrived home at 4.30pm to a lovely welcome home from Nicola and the children, and then I slumped into the armchair – who thought being the passenger in a car could be so exhausting? It's great to be back but although I am on 'home turf' I can't help feeling very disoriented. ZZZZ.

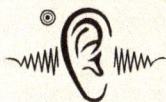

Back to life.
Back to reality.

21st May (8 DAYS POST OP)

I woke up early after a restless night. I have to sleep almost sitting straight up so couldn't get comfortable, and this disturbs my wife too.

Even though my home surroundings are familiar, I have to rely on others being with me to get around. I can walk unaided but have to do so looking straight ahead and very slowly. I am unable to look up or down or side to side. I spent most of today sat on the sofa but I find too much sitting around gives me backache. I had a nap in the afternoon. I find my eye is still drying up but more noticeably when I am tired. Nicola helped me into the bath – it's good to have a nice long soak at last.

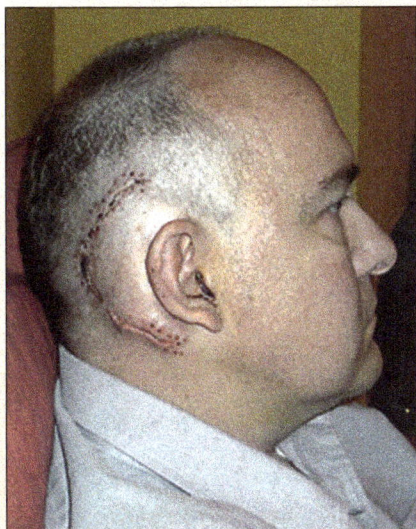

22nd May (9 DAYS POST OP)

Another restless night, although Nicola has let me have the double bed to myself then she can get a good night's sleep at least. I can't relax, and I can only spend a short time watching TV or sitting in the garden, or on the computer.

I feel very fidgety. I am also struggling to come to terms with the deafness. I notice it more at home when there is a lot of activity – children playing, TV on, people in the kitchen. I think it'll take some getting used to. Friends called this afternoon, and when they were leaving, I walked around the block with them. This is my first time outside since returning and it felt a little disconcerting as I can still only walk in a straight line.

23rd May (10 DAYS POST OP)

Nicola & the children went out this morning for a couple of hours and left me to my own devices – I survived! Seem to be moving around the house a little easier, don't feel as restricted although still tentative of my surroundings. My dry eye is still a bother to me, and I have to wet it occasional with 'hypo tears' and I tape it up at night. I managed to venture into the loft today, where my study is located. First time up ladders (& down).

24th May (11 DAYS POST OP)

I awoke after a better night although still not totally undisturbed. We drove to Ulverston (10 minutes away), and we had a stroll to the bank. I had no need for pills to prevent car sickness but took them just in case. It felt strange walking down a busy (and cobbled) street for the first time, but I was guided well. I was quite surprised at how tired this jaunt made me feel and I fell asleep on the sofa early evening.

25th May (12 DAYS POST OP)

We ventured out to Barrow-in-Furness this afternoon and had our lunch out. Afterwards we did a little shopping in the town centre – I handled it like a pro! I am getting less fazed by such outings every day.

26th May (13 DAYS POST OP)

The nights are starting to get a little more restful, although I still can't get comfortable or sleep all through yet. I am beginning to relax more and can work at the computer for longer periods which stimulates the brain cells. I went to the supermarket for the weekly shop. Pushed the trolley round and loaded some of the lighter bags.

When the children came home from school we walked to the in-laws ... around a quarter of mile away, furthest I've walked yet, and can feel my self confidence growing. My walking is becoming more animated, less robotic and I can now even look from side to side.

This evening I went to ASDA with in-laws which is my first trip out without first time out without the missus to guide me. I was overwhelmed by the noise in the supermarket – it is the first crowded place I have been to and I couldn't stand it for too long. It felt good to be doing more but I am aware of the fact that I shouldn't do too much as there is still a risk of fluid leakage if too much is done too soon.

27th May (14 DAYS POST OP)

It is now a fortnight since the operation and one week since I came home. I am still experiencing disturbed nights, I can't get comfortable. I can sleep on my back for a while, then on my 'good' side, then propped up in bed but nothing seems to give comfort – I even tried briefly on my bad side, but it's not ready to be slept on yet.

My eye gives me a little discomfort and has to be wet periodically and when I eat or drink I have a tendency to dribble or bite my inner lip because I can't open my mouth wide enough.

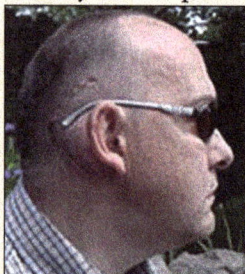

The upper part of the scar is healing nicely and has a lovely scab on it. The photo shows how the scar is doing. My hearing is taking some getting used to, and I have tinnitus in the bad ear, which is like a constant annoying washing machine.

30th May (17 DAYS POST OP)

I am now sleeping a lot easier. I can lie on my back and left side with just a single pillow, so I am sleeping almost the night through. My eye is still causing me discomfort, but the children have found me a pirate eye patch that I wear to alleviate the situation. I can move around a lot easier and even managed to kick a football to the children in the park today. I feel very dizzy if I close my eyes while moving so this is still a problem. The scabs on my scar are starting to come off now also – very nice.

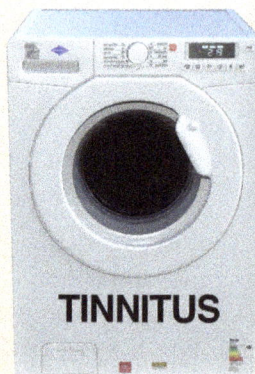

TINNITUS

4rd June (22 DAYS POST OP)

It is getting increasingly comfortable to sleep all the way through the night; I don't feel as restless and find I can concentrate more easily during the day. I awoke with a terrible pain in my lower spine. I decided to go to the doctors to make sure it wasn't related to spinal fluid leakage – it turned out to be a pulled muscle.

I read an online survey of post-A.N. operation problems and 25% experienced CSF leakage post-op, so it has got me a little paranoid I think. CSF leakage can lead to infections such as severe meningitis. Funnily enough, the exercise of walking to the surgery made my back feel better anyway! The wife and kids are going away today for the weekend to a wedding, so I am to have a friend stay and 'babysit'. I am feeling much better and growing accustomed to my loss of hearing. My 'get up and go' is slowly rising to its wobbly feet, and my overall confidence is blooming

5th June (23 DAYS POST OP)

I went for a walk with my 'babysitter' and his children this afternoon. The boys took their bicycles. To test my balance I had a sit on the eldest boy's bike and I rode it for a short distance (very slowly, close to grass in case I needed to jump off) and to my amazement, I kept my balance – I didn't think I would be able to ride a bike for some time to come.

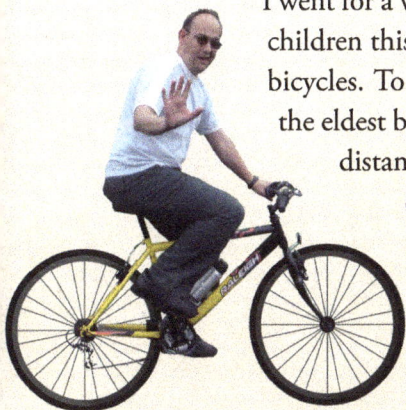

Also today I received yet another reassuring letter in the post from Prof. Ramsden, to confirm the tumour was benign and I wouldn't have to return to the hospital for any form of cancer treatment.

Children's University Hospitals

NHS Trust

Department of Otolaryngology - Head and Neck Surgery
Manchester Royal Infirmary
Oxford Road
Manchester
M13 9W

Professor Ramsden's secretary:

Typed: 25 May 04

Mr Russell Holden

Dear Mr Holden

This is just to let you know that the tumour we recently removed from your head examined by the pathologists. They confirmed that this was a normal aco neuroma with no evidence of malignancy.

Yours sincerely

Professor R T Ramsden
Professor of Otolaryngology

17th June (36 DAYS POST OP)

Things are improving daily. When I think that is was only a month ago since the operation, I can't believe how my body has adapted in just a short time.

The hearing in my right ear has gone permanently – I know it will never return and single-sided deafness has taken some getting used to. I notice it more in crowded places, but my friends are starting to remember to come to my hearing side if they need to speak to me.

One aspect of impaired hearing on one side is that I find I have difficulty determining the direction of sounds. This can make it dangerous to cross a street or otherwise navigate in traffic. The most common symptom is an inability to separate background noise from the sounds I want to hear. It's like a lack of depth perception of noise instead of sight.

For those who have not experienced single-sided deafness, it is difficult to appreciate the handicaps presented and the lifestyle changes that occur for this type of hearing loss. Many patients learn to live with a unilateral hearing loss. Others have to make significant life changes as they may feel highly uncomfortable and no longer easily able to cope in everyday environments, such as business meetings, busy restaurants or family gatherings.

My balance hasn't been affected as much as I had anticipated. I can't walk in a straight line yet, but I can move my head from side to side without falling over.

I am driving again – which is excellent news. In fact, it is easier to drive than to be a passenger as my deaf ear is towards the driver's door, and I can hear what is going on in the car.

I still have a little trouble with my right eye drying up. I have drops and gel from the doctor, but I find wearing spectacles beneficial (I previously only had to wear them for driving, but find I can wear them all the time now). I've been told of an operation that implants small weights in the eyelid to assist them in closing, but I don't think I need this. My good sleep pattern has returned I am pleased to say, and I can sleep on my right side now too (although my ear still feels prosthetic).

The doctor says I may be able to return to work next month. Pre-op I had been a graphic designer at a printing firm. I also had a self-employed cleaning business, which I had to sell due to the amount of time I would be away from work during my recovery. Now I need to start looking for a new career to accommodate my 'disabilities', which at age 38 is both a daunting and exciting prospect.

Over the past few weeks, My family and friends have been marvellous support, Nicola was there for me when I needed her most. For this, I will always be grateful.

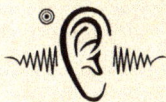

Facing the future

Today is the appointment for my four weeks check-up. This is my first return to Manchester Royal Infirmary since the operation. After a short wait, I was called in to see the consultant, Mr Kevin Green.

He was a nice chap, and we discussed how I had been coping with going home. He did some balance tests with me and checked inside my ear. He recommended I take another two months off work and continue to avoid heavy lifting, strenuous activity and swimming.

I told him I am feeling much better and eager to get more active, he explained that though this was a good sign of my recovery, I should view this time of enforced inactivity as a part of the healing process. He also pointed out that things hadn't fully healed at the operation site; thus, there was still a danger of CSF leaks occurring. Fair enough! I thanked him for his advice and made an appointment to see him again on the 23rd of August.

Two more months off work – this time last year I would have loved to have had two months summer vacation, but this means by then I will have been out of a work routine for almost six months in total. I sold my business due to ill health back in March. I have worked continually for the past 22 years with no time off for sickness and average vacation times each year, so this is a marathon for me. I need the routine of work, and I hate relying on the state for my income. I never thought I'd say it but I can't wait to get back into the rat race! *(This period was during the height of the Euro 2004 soccer tournament and the Wimbledon fortnight – a time many people would love to have spent at home with access to a TV and a fridge – however, I am not a sports fan wahhhh!).*

9th July (8 WEEKS AND 1 DAY POST OP)

It is now eight weeks post-operation – I can't believe it has been that long since the Acoustic Neuroma was removed.

The progress that I have made is incredible. My sleep pattern has recovered totally, and I no longer have disturbed nights now, I can lie on my right side. My right ear is still protruding more than the left side – I often wonder if it was sewn back in the correct position, after all, during the operation I was lying on my left ear, so there was no point of reference!

I no longer wake with a headache or for that matter with the awful facial pain that has haunted me for the past seven years. I can walk in a straight line, but in low light or when I close my eyes I go a little off course (but how often do you close your eyes when you go for a walk?). Strangely enough, when I have had a glass of wine, this side effect is emphasised even more!

My hair has grown well since the operation and has covered the operation site – the scar has healed up nicely too. My face is still paralysed on the right side although this is showing signs of movement – I can do a faint smile with a half-cocked eyebrow, but only if I concentrate! My eye still dries up, but this is most apparent on warm, breezy days. The consultant I saw last week advised me to continue to tape my eyelid down at night – I hate doing this, not that it is unpleasant to have tape holding the eyelid down, it is the pulling off in the morning that is the worst part!

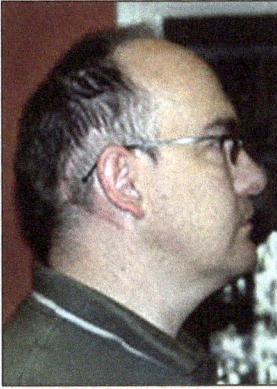

My eyes seem to more sensitive to light than before the operation, so I use photochromic spectacles now most of the time. My taste-buds haven't fully returned yet – what an unusual side effect, to lose part of your sense of taste. Also, I quite often bite my lip because the right side of the mouth doesn't open fully – this is most annoying as any bite always becomes like a mouth ulcer and then takes a painful week to go away. My energy is returning daily. I have been putting my enforced time off to good use and been attending college courses for two mornings a week to improve Photoshop skills and learning HTML and web design which has been beneficial. I am feeling positive about the future; I can see a way forward and even though it is an ill-defined 'forward' which like me staggers a little at times I know it is forward and not a backwards step.

12th August (12 WEEKS POST OP)

Three months have now passed since the surgery. The time has flown by – yet on another level, it seems like a lifetime ago. I continue to make progress. I now feel about 95% fit and can do many of the things I could do before the operation – although a little more cautiously. I sleep OK now, and I have no headaches or facial pain. My face is becoming more expressive. I am not on any medication of any kind and have not needed any since May. This has been great for me as I had depended on taking pain killers regularly for the past couple of years to combat my facial pains – I don't miss them or the side-effects.

I hate to be in crowded areas – the loss of hearing on my right side is very disconcerting, and for the first time in my life, I can understand how someone could get a panic attack in certain situations. Although my balance hasn't been as affected as anticipated.

I feel like my centre of balance has altered rather than losing it. I have a few problems with it, but this is usually confined to getting a bit wobbly on uneven ground. Despite this, I have had a good summer, and it hasn't stopped me being active, especially with both children off school, and my recovery has gone relatively smoothly.

As you can see from the picture, my face is still a bit expressionless on the right side, and my eyelid stays open most of the time. My scar has healed nicely though, and my hair has now grown over it, so it is covered up.

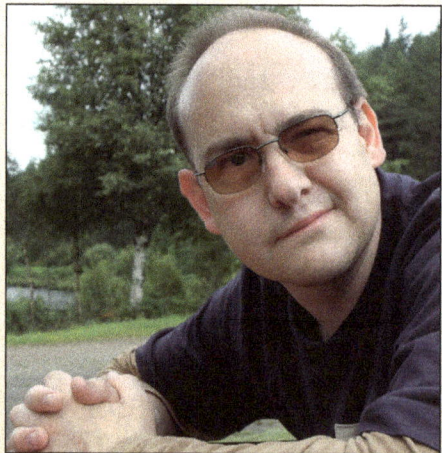

25th August (3 MONTHS, 2 WEEKS POST OP)

My three-month check-up was changed from Monday to Wednesday this week, so once again we made the trip to Manchester Royal Infirmary. We found it the first time without getting lost or taking a wrong turning! In the ENT waiting room, I bumped into Kevin Cheung, who assisted Prof. Ramsden with my operation, he was pleased to see the progress I had made – he's an amiable chap. I then saw Mr Green, who did the usual tests; "Close your eyes, frown, open & close your mouth, raise your eyebrows, etc." and was happy with my progress too. He could see real improvement in my facial movement. He told me I was eligible for a bone-anchored hearing aid (Baha®) – this would help me distinguish noise coming from the deaf side. I will find out more when I return for the next appointment in November. Mr Green said I was now fit enough to return to work.

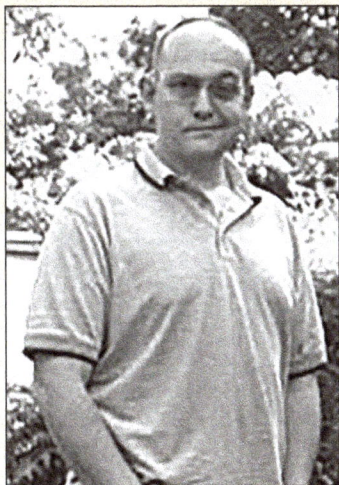

The following day I saw my own G.P. and got my final 'sick note' which expires on the 1st Sept. I have decided to become self-employed again so I'm starting up a new business offering graphic design and short-run printing services aimed at small businesses, or individuals who don't want the expense of big minimum print runs. I am also starting a part time Foundation degree course in New Media from next month at UCLAN.

10th October (JUST UNDER 5 MONTHS POST OP)

Here we are looking at almost half a year since the operation, and I continue to make rapid progress. Just looking through these pages reminds me of how bad I was and how much things have progressed. I met some friends last weekend who haven't seen me since they visited me in the hospital and they couldn't believe the improvement in my facial movement. With every week that passes the paralysis subsides.

I can now smile, raise an eyebrow and whistle a happy tune. I can walk in a straight line and ride my bicycle without any difficulty (although if I look over my shoulder when riding, I find myself veering to the right without realising!). I started work on the 1st of September – my design and print business is going well, and I'm building a good client base. However, I found myself doing too much too soon. I launched myself into a busy schedule from day one but soon realised I don't have the same stamina for work that I used to have pre-op. I have to 'pace' myself and just do enough to prevent myself from getting worn out.

11th December (7 MONTHS POST OP)

Another month, another season – things are still going fine, I feel as well as I have been in a long while – not having the awful facial pain that had afflicted my days before the operation is great, this is the first time in seven years I have not been in agony every other month. The two things I have noticed about the aftermath of the operation in winter are:

> 1. I feel less coordinated in the dark, and because the days are much shorter, I find this has affected me more in the winter months than in the summer.

2. I feel the cold more on my head – I have always been follically challenged, but have never felt the chilly weather on my head so much as this year – especially around the operation site. It's no big deal, and I do have a hat.

Everything else is slowly returning to some normality. The hearing loss will of course always be with me, and I still find this to be the biggest handicap. I find that I only hear about 80% of what is said to me, and in a crowded room that goes down to 40% at best. The hospital cancelled my next check-up. It should have been in November, but it is now February.

12th April 2005 (11 MONTHS POST OP)

Well, things have certainly moved on since the last entry in the journal – I am now looking at almost 12 months since the operation and boy has my life changed in that time.

When I last updated the diary five months ago in December, I was waiting for a job interview. You may recall I started a design & print business last September. Although the work was steadily increasing, I could foresee it being some time before it was a reliable wage earner. I decided to keep an eye on the employment section in the local newspapers. One job caught my eye – for a Graphic Designer in the Marketing department at a local book publisher. I applied for the situation, was accepted for an interview and got the job! I started in January and have just completed my first 12 weeks.

This time last year, I was facing a potentially life-threatening ailment with the prospect of a major operation and recovery time and no concrete post-op employment plans. I am amazed at my improvement. If anyone reading this diary is worried about life after Acoustic Neuroma surgery, then I can testify that although it isn't an easy or pleasant experience, by remaining positive your recovery will be less of a burden.

The only lasting regret that I have is my hearing loss, and while for 50% of the time, it isn't a problem the other 50% is more difficult to cope with. I have become more insular, more unsociable because I know that I can't hear what is being said so I avoid social situations. The only way to get more from these occasions will be to acquire a hearing aid, but my choices are limited because of the single-sided deafness and the fact there is nothing to amplify on that side anyway.

Styles of Hearing Aids

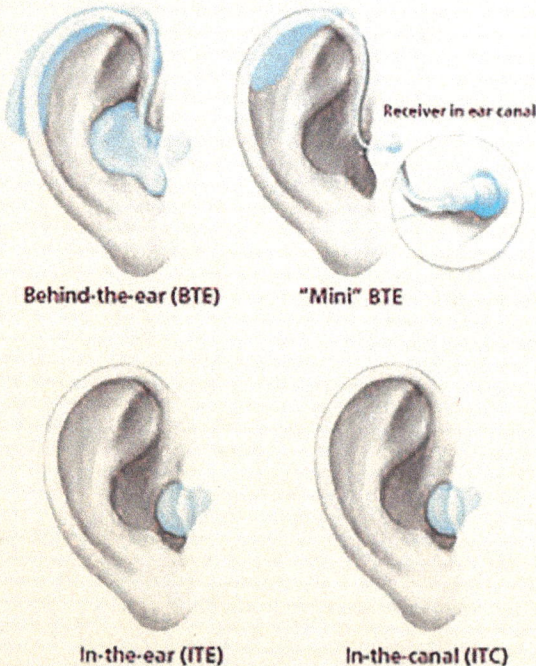

NH Medical Arts

Receiver in ear canal

Behind-the-ear (BTE)   "Mini" BTE

In-the-ear (ITE)   In-the-canal (ITC)

I have an appointment to see the Baha® people next month but as the whole procedure (from initial assessment to the day the thing is up and running and usable) could take 18 months and involves further surgery around an already sensitive operation site, I don't think I can be bothered with the hassle. I need a hearing aid that I can quickly put on in certain situations then stick back in my pocket. Even if this means wearing something the size of a tennis ball, at least it means I won't miss out as much.

My face is still partially paralysed, and it is only when I make big facial gestures that others notice there has been a problem. I have developed a 'dint' in my chin and was wondering if this is through muscle wastage on that side.

It has certainly been an 'interesting' year and has gone by very quickly. I can't wait to see what Year 2 brings!

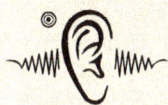

One year on

13th May 2005 (12 MONTHS POST OP)

Twelve months ago I had an operation that has changed my life. If I had a snapshot of my life today back then, I wouldn't have recognised myself.

The past year has been a roller coaster of mixed experiences for me, like a baby taking its first steps there are things I could do before that I'll never be able to do again and there are things that I can do that I didn't think would ever be possible.

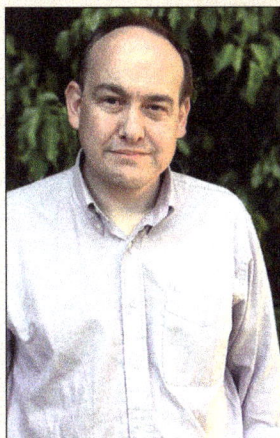

12 months post op

Profile of my life now

HEARING – On the Right side it will never return, but on the left side it is as good as ever. Late last year I went to a rock concert – big mistake, my 'good' ear was ringing for days after and it made me realise I have to look after this side as a future investment. I have, as time progresses, got more used to being in crowded rooms. I am learning to sift out the noises I hear and realise my limitations. In years to come, I may need to get a Baha® hearing aid, and I intend to get lip-reading lessons soon.

BALANCE – This hasn't been as much a problem as I thought it would be. I only notice it when I am tired, and I stumble occasionally, but I don't experience dizzy spells or nausea. I haven't been on any fairground rides, on a ship or done roly-polies since the operation so I don't know how I'd be in these situations, but I'll keep you posted when they happen.

FACIAL PARALYSIS – My face has not returned to its previous animated state although it is better than it was. I can't open my mouth fully on the right side, and I can't raise my right eyebrow. My taste buds haven't fully got their taste back yet either.

My eyelids both blink now – quite often at the same time! If I blink fast though both lids don't work at the same time. The right eye still gets dry and crusty.

IN GENERAL – I find I get tired by evening time. My get up & go quickly gets up and sprints off. I am always ready for my bed.

Also, you know that feeling when you have a word you want to say 'on the tip of your tongue' and no matter how hard you concentrate it just won't come out? I have never been the most eloquent of speakers but since the operation I find it difficult to express myself as instantly as I'd like. This is a better explanation of it ...

The tip-of-the-tongue phenomenon, (sometimes called "presque vu" – almost seen), is the failure to retrieve a word from memory, combined with partial recall and the feeling that retrieval is imminent. The phenomenon's name comes from the saying, "It's on the tip of my tongue." The tip of the tongue phenomenon reveals that lexical access occurs in stages.

People experiencing the tip-of-the-tongue phenomenon can often recall one or more features of the target word, such as the first letter, its syllabic stress, and words similar in sound and/or meaning. Individuals report a feeling of being seized by the state, feeling something like mild anguish while searching for the word, and a sense of relief when the word is found. While many aspects of the tip-of-the-tongue state remain unclear, there are two major competing explanations for its occurrence, the direct-access view and the inferential view. The direct-access view posits that the state occurs when memory strength is not enough to recall an item, but is strong enough to trigger the state. The inferential view claims that Tip-of-the-tongues aren't completely based on inaccessible, yet activated targets; rather they arise when the rememberer tries to piece together different clues about the word. Emotional-induced retrieval often causes more Tip-of-the-tongue experiences than an emotionally neutral retrieval, such as asking where a famous icon was assassinated rather than simply asking the capital city of a state. Emotional Tip-of-the-tongue experiences also have a longer retrieval time than non-emotional Tip-of-the-tongue experiences. The cause of this is unknown but possibilities include using a different retrieval strategy when having an emotional Tip-of-the-tongue experience rather than a non-emotional Tip-of-the-tongue experience, fluency at the time of retrieval, and strength of memory.

Tip-of-the-tongue states should be separated from 'feeling-of-knowing' (feeling of knowing) states. 'feeling-of-knowing', in contrast, is the feeling that one will be able to recognise - from a list of items - an item that is currently inaccessible. There are still currently opposing articles of the separability of the process underlying these concepts. However there is some evidence that Tip-of-the-tongues and 'feeling-of-knowing's draw on different parts of the brain. Tip-of-the-tongues are associated with the anterior cingulate, right dorsolateral pre-frontal cortex, and right inferior cortex while 'feeling-of-knowing's are not.

An occasional tip-of-the-tongue state is normal for people of all ages. Tip-of-the-tongue becomes more frequent as people age. Tip-of-the-tongue is only a medical condition when it becomes frequent enough to interfere with learning or daily life. This disorder is called anomic aphasia when acquired by brain damage, usually from a head injury, stroke, or dementia.

My social life has been affected – because I can't hear well in crowds (i.e. groups of more than two!!) Or if there is much background noise (i.e. louder than a pin dropping). Even walking down the street is difficult with so much background street related noise to contend with. I find it hard to interact. I tend to miss part of what is being said and end up asking the questions people have just answered or just end up nodding or agreeing with what people are saying.

On a positive note – I am still here. The tumour was touching my brain stem before removal so if it hadn't been detected when it was, I could be lying in a coma right now ... or worse.

I am grateful for my life, and even though I have had a little moan on these pages about how my life has been affected these past twelve months, I have written these things as a personal diary, as part of the healing process. I know there are many people out there experiencing far worse ailments and treatments and prognosis that make what I have gone through look like a walk in the park. I wrote these things to try and put a positive spin on things, to show anyone facing the same operation that there is life after Acoustic Neuroma, that even though certain aspects of our life as we know it ends the moment our tumour is removed, it certainly doesn't mean we can't enjoy a full life post-op.

In the past year I have started a small business, enrolled at the local university, got a job at the UK's most successful educational book publishers and bought a little red sporty car to commute to work in.

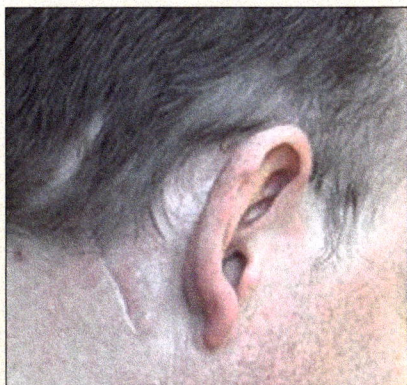

Twelve months on, the scar has healed well

These things are achievements but are secondary to the things I would have missed had I not been here – listening to my wife play the piano, sharing a funny moment with my son or helping my little girl ride her bike without stabilisers.

So here is to the future. I'll continue to update this diary – although perhaps not as often. The time has come to stop looking at the past, at what I used to have or be able to do and concentrate on what I am now able to do and learn to live within my limitations but develop my strengths.

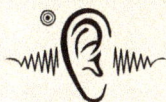

There is more

Two years have now passed since the operation to remove the tumour (and over 12 months since the last diary entry). Looking back over that time I can honestly say it has been the single most empowering period of my life so far.

The first year was spent getting physically fit – getting used to the disabilities & learning my limitations in various situations.

The second year was I think the most significant as it has shaped the person I have now (and continue to) become. Almost a year to the day after the operation I was hit by a tidal wave of emotions – to call it post-traumatic stress would be too strong but something very similar hit me like a smack in the face.

Two years on

I was suddenly consumed with "What ifs"... What if the doctor hadn't found the tumour when he did? What if something had gone wrong during the long operation? What if? What if? What if? ...

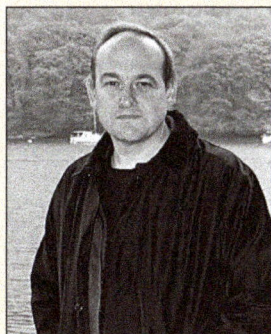

63

I began to really examine my life, where my true values lay and what mattered to me most. My family had been there for me during the whole episode ... from diagnosis, to operation, to recovery and beyond – they showed an unconditional love that I found was lacking in some so-called friends.

Also for months I had noticed cognitive issues, I find it harder to retain information, I find I have to take notes now at work to remind myself of procedures. If I need to remember to take something out with me I have to leave it by the front door or I will simply forget! I have read though that these things are not uncommon amongst post-op patients so at least I am in good company. Will it get any better ... only time will tell.

I recently found an article which convinced me I wasn't alone with these cognitive flaws:

> *'Those who treated me told me that I would probably experience short term memory problems. That was verified during countless neuropsychological tests. My short term memory loss was evaluated at a 10% loss. After my AN surgery, I endured many tests, some of which were neuropsychological tests. The bottom line result was that I had lost a significant % of IQ and at least 10% of my short term memory. That helped me to understand why I couldn't remember so many thing such as prior to discovery of the AN... I've had to change my lifestyle and profession.'*

www.anarchive.org/cognitive

Profile of my life now

HEARING – I have recently started lip-reading classes to help with communication problems. I find it a useful exercise, and it's good to spend time with others in the same boat. I attend a weekly class at the local Age Concern - a magnet for the hard of hearing! It's great fun at the classes spending time with the older generation and drinking tea. Lip reading isn't as easy to pick up as you might think – especially when you have some hearing. The sounds distract. I suppose it's like a person who is blind in one eye learning Braille - it's an excellent skill to learn and helps to a certain degree, but until your life depends on that skill it is harder to build the same enthusiasm. I decided not to go for a Baha® hearing aid as I explained previously, but I am investigating CROS hearing aids at the moment to see if they would be of benefit.

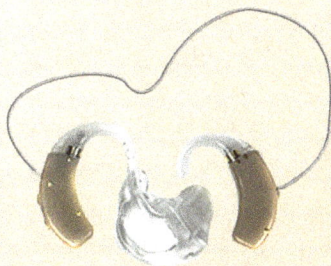

CROS hearing aids

A Contralateral Routing of Signals – or CROS – hearing system is used for people who have one normally hearing ear and one deaf or unaidable ear. The unaidable ear has a microphone transmitting to a receiver in the normal ear, which therefore picks up sound from both sides of the wearer.

As the month's pass, my deafness is less of an issue – I have grown more accustomed to it, as have my family. People automatically walk on my 'good side', I know where best to position myself when we go to a restaurant, and which places I feel most happy & confident visiting.

BALANCE – I sometimes carry a walking pole around with me. I find on certain terrain, rough ground or slopes that I am quite unsteady. During a recent period of snow I had it with me all the time as I found the slippery pavements very challenging.

FACIAL PARALYSIS – As each year passes I see some return to previous form. My eye still gets crusty but usually more so at night when I am tired or when it is windy ... It's not a big problem though.

IN GENERAL – I don't get as tired as I did 12 months ago but I find I get 'suddenly tired' – it's as if I get to a certain point then switch off rather than a progressive winding down.

I am still plagued by tinnitus. At times worse than others but I have again grown accustomed to it. It is the washing machine type which rumbles on quietly in the background.

MENTAL HEALTH – I was much more positive this time last year. The past 12 months have been a voyage of discovery, I have suffered depression for the first time in my life and have made radical changes to my life. And I stepped away from the religion I have been a member of for the past 30 years. I seem to be 'between lives' at this time, and I am both excited and scared to see what the future holds.

I am still grateful to be here, I have a wife, 2 brilliant children, a fantastic family and working as a Graphic Designer for an educational book publishers in the Lake District so I have every reason to be thankful.

A couple of additions...

I have recently taken possession of a set of CROS hearing aids. There is one for each ear. The one in the 'bad' ear is a micro-phone that picks up sound on the deaf side and sends it via the wire that connects them to the 'good' ear which is basically a speaker. Both aids fit snugly in the ears and are relatively comfortable to wear. My quality of life has increased dramatically since I got them. I no longer feel claus-trophobic when in crowded or noisy areas and I can even posi-tion myself between people when out for a walk and keep up with

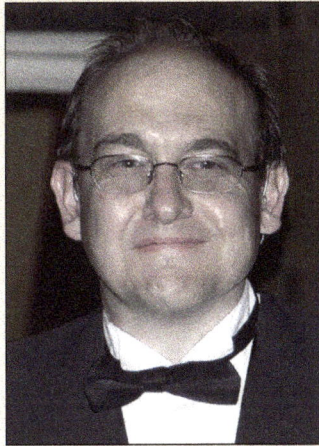
Wearing my CROS hearing aids at a charity function

the conversation! It is certainly no substitute for 'real ears' but is a very good alternative.

Also...

In June (2006) I had my yearly MRI scan and the results were good – no sign of regrowth of my tumour and everything has healed up nicely. I have my final appointment at Manchester Royal Infirmary booked for next week (Nov 4th 2006) – 2 years 5 months 20 days post-op!) And I have been told it will be my last and that I will be officially discharged. Thus another chapter in this saga comes to an end!

In 2007 the family and I joined a local amateur drama group and appeared in pantomime – this was a great achievement for me. Despite being deaf, having dodgy balance and becoming self conscious since the operation I regained confidence by performing on a stage (for fun).

Thank you for continuing to listen to my ramblings, I hope you have not found it too boring and if anyone would like to contact me about your own experience feel free to do so. I will keep you posted!!

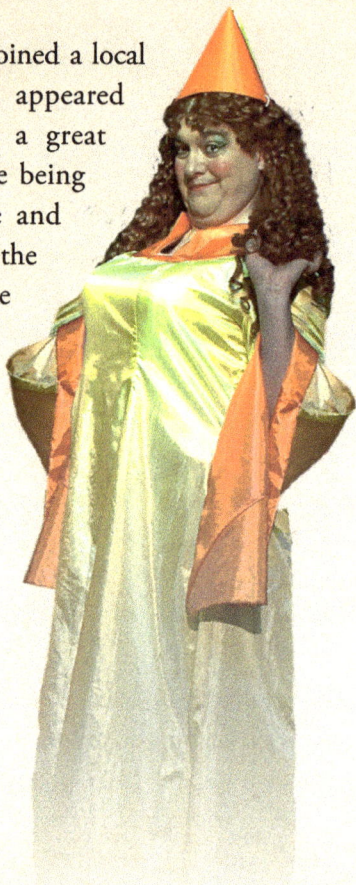

Honeysuckle, a very ugly sister!

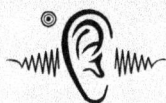

That was to be last post I made on the diary blog. A couple of years later the free Yahoo web hosting I was using ended and the site went offline.

The story didn't end there though – even though I thought it had! Over the next few years my life course would change in ways I couldn't imagine including an addition to the legacy left by acoustic neuroma.

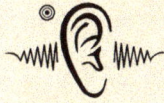

One Decade Later

It is now (at the time of writing) May 2016, which is now twelve years post-op ... TWELVE YEARS! Where has the time gone?

To recap ... in 2006 when I last made an entry in the diary I was working for an Educational Publishing Company, I had a young family and had recently taken possession of a set of CROS hearing aids. Apart from the after-effects of the operation I've mentioned several times so far, I experienced no more problems, re-occurrences or medical issues associated with the Acoustic Neuroma.

Life continued it's normal routine for the next few years then...

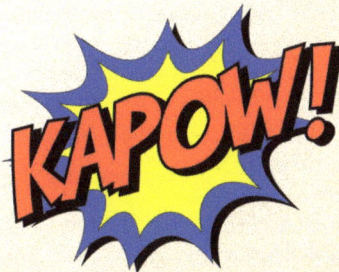

In 2008, after 18 years together, Nicola and I decided to go our separate ways and we had an amicable divorce in 2009.

I was on my own for a short while, then just over 12 months later I got married to Sharon.

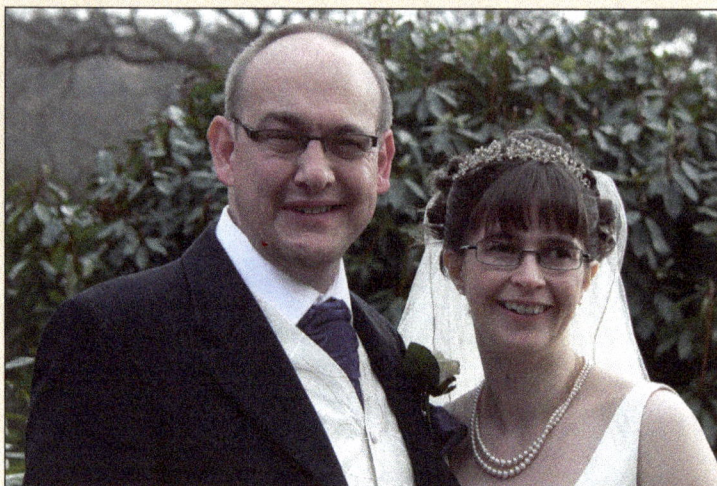

By December 2010 Sharon was 6 months pregnant and on a visit to the hospital for a check-up, we had to go via the ENT department. I thought I'd take the opportunity to pop in for some batteries for the CROS hearing aids which I still occasionally used and arranged to meet Sharon after her appointment.

Whilst in ENT I bumped into a chap from the Audiology department who had fitted my hearing aids back in 2006. He invited me into his room for a chat about current hearing aids and upgrade options. During the course of the conversation he asked if I'd ever considered a Bone Anchored Hearing Aid ... I told him I'd been offered a Baha® shortly after the operation in 2004.

Back then the wound was still fresh, and I'd had enough of operations and hospitals, plus because the procedure had to be done in Manchester, it would mean a four hour and 200 miles round trip every appointment.

The audiologist told me the good news was that the operation was now available locally, there at Furness General Hospital the very hospital where we now sat in Barrow-in-Furness, just 8 miles from my home.

I made an appointment to return and took away some leaflets about Baha® with me to investigate the possibility and make some important decisions.

PROS	CONS
• Improved hearing • Convenient • Ease of use • Small • No wires • Accessories	• Operation required to install • Regular chance of Infection • Self concious • Physical Activity Limitations • Irritation • Possibility of Loss • Not waterproof

I was offered the use of an 'Alice band'. This is a simple hair-band with a hearing aid attached to it that presses against the skull and give the same effect, although not quite as clear, as one anchored directly into the bone.

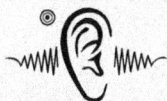

Bone Anchored Hearing
a short history

Bone-anchored hearing aids use a surgically implanted abutment to transmit sound by direct conduction through bone to the inner ear, by-passing the external auditory canal and middle ear. A titanium prosthesis is surgically embedded into the skull with a small abutment exposed outside the skin. A sound processor sits on this abutment and transmits sound vibrations to the titanium implant. The implant vibrates the skull and inner ear, which stimulate the nerve fibers of the inner ear, allowing hearing.

The surgery is often performed under local anaesthesia and as an outpatient procedure. An important piece of information for patients is that if they for whatever reason are not satisfied with the BAHA solution, removing the implant is easy. No other ear surgical procedure is reversible like this.

By bypassing the outer or middle ear, BAHA can increase hearing in noisy situations and help localise sounds. In addition to improved speech understanding, it results in a natural sound with less distortion and feedback compared with conventional hearing aids. The ear canal is left open for comfort, and helps to reduce any problems caused by chronic ear infections or allergies. In patients with single-sided sensorineural deafness,

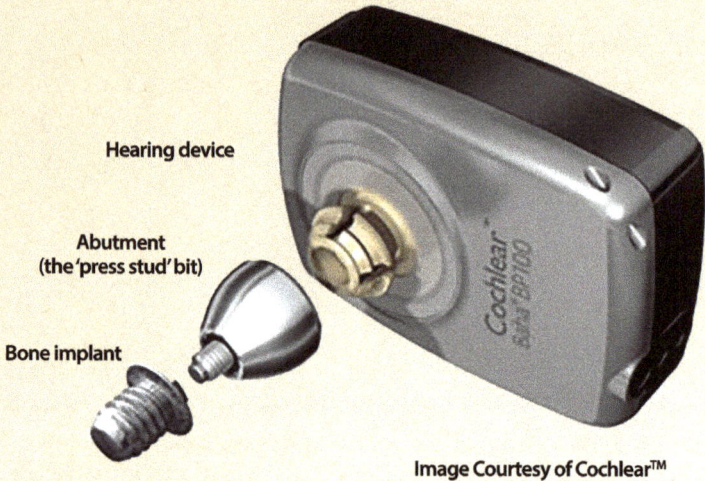

Hearing device

Abutment
(the 'press stud' bit)

Bone implant

Image Courtesy of Cochlear™

BAHA sends the sound by the skull bone from the deaf side to the inner ear of the hearing side. This transfer of sound gives a 360° sound awareness.

Single-sided deafness

A person with unilateral hearing loss may have functional difficulty hearing even when the other ear is normal, particularly in demanding situations such as noisy environments and when several people are speaking the same time. A complication in single-sided deafness is hearing impairment in the hearing ear. Conventional ear surgery involves a risk of hearing loss due to the surgical procedure. Most ear surgeons are thus reluctant to perform surgery on an only hearing ear. The BAHA surgery avoids this risk and may be an appropriate treatment. An extended trial of a BAHA system with a headband prior to surgery led to more realistic expectations. In the trial, 50% of the candidates wished to proceed to surgery.

Complications of BAHA systems can be considered as either related to the bone (hard tissue) or the soft tissue.

Bone

- Failure of osseointegration
- Chronic infection
- Trauma

Soft tissue

- Irritation of the skin surrounding the implant
- Death of the skin flap
- Overgrowth of skin over the device
- Wound dehiscence (splitting apart of the wound)
- Bleeding or hematoma formation
- Persistent pain

Soft-tissue complications are much more common, and most are managed with topical treatments. Children are more likely to suffer both kinds of complications than adults. Sometimes, a second surgical procedure is required. Complications are less likely with good wound hygiene. Other drawbacks of BAHA include accidental or spontaneous loss of the bone implant, and patient refusal for treatment due to stigma.

Surgical procedure

The bone behind the ear is exposed through a U-shaped or straight incision or with the help of a specially designed BAHA dermatome. A hole, 3 or 4 mm deep depending on the thickness of the bone, is drilled. The hole is widened and the implant with the mounted coupling is inserted under generous cooling to minimize surgical trauma to the bone.

Some surgeons perform a reduction of the subcutaneous soft tissue. The rationale for this is to reduce the mobility between implant and skin to avoid inflammation at the penetration site. This reduction of the soft tissue has been questioned and some surgeons do not perform any or a minimum of it. The rationale for this is that any surgery will result in some scar tissue that could be the focus of infection. The infections seen early during the development of the surgical procedure could perhaps be explained by the lack of seal between implant and abutment allowing bacteria to enter the space. A new helium tight seal may be advantageous and prevent biofilm formation. This will also allow the surgeon to use longer abutments should a need exist. Three to six weeks later or even earlier, the audiologist will fit and adjust the hearing processor according to the patient's hearing level. The fitting will be made using a special program in a computer.

Handling

An area where skin is penetrated requires care and cleaning because of the risk of inflammation around the abutment. Daily cleaning is required.

History

Patients with chronic ear infection where the drum and/or the small bones in the middle ear are damaged often have hearing loss, but difficulties in using a hearing aid fitted in the ear canal. Direct bone conduction through a vibrator attached to a skin-penetrating implant addresses these disadvantages.

In 1977, the first three patients were implanted with a bone-conduction hearing solution by Anders Tjellström at the Ear, Nose, and Throat Department at Sahlgrenska University

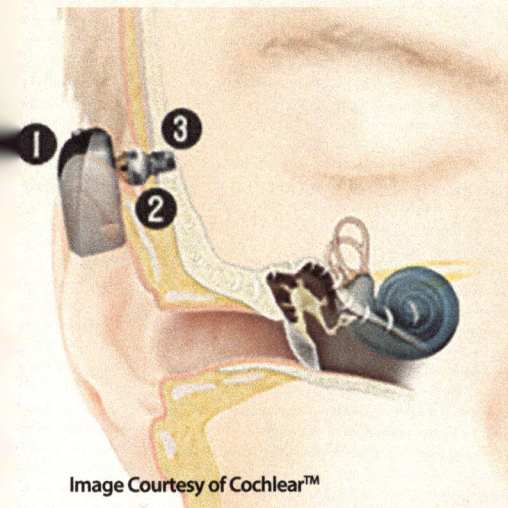

Image Courtesy of Cochlear™

How the system works

A small titanium implant sits in the bone behind your ear.

Attached to the implant is an abutment that extends just above the skin.

The sound processor fits onto the abutment to hold it in place.

Sound travels as vibrations from the processor via the abutment to the implant, which then directs the vibrations through the bone to stimulate the inner ear.

1. Sound processor
2. Abutment
3. Implant

Hospital in Gothenburg, Sweden. A 4-mm-long titanium screw with a diameter of 3.75 mm was inserted in the bone behind the ear, and a bone conduction hearing aid was attached. The term osseointegration was coined by Professor Brånemark. During animal studies, he found the bone tissue attached to the titanium implant without any soft tissue in between. He also showed an such an implant could take a heavy load. His definition of osseointegration was "direct contact between living bone and an implant that can take a load".

The first clinical application of titanium was in oral surgery, where implants were used for retention of dentures. Brånemark sought an acoustic way to evaluate osseointegration. A patient with implants in the jaws was fitted with a bone vibrator on one of his implants. When tested, the patient experienced very loud sound even at low stimulation levels, indicating sound could propagate very well in the bone. It has later been shown by Håkansson that the sound transmission in bone is linear, indicating low distortion of the sound.

The implant in the bone is made of titanium and will osse-ointegrate. The hearing instrument is impedance-matched. Osseointegration has been defined as the direct contact between living bone and an implant that can take a load, with no soft tissue at the interface.

Costs

In the US, the cost of the Baha device is about $4,000. The cost of the titanium implant, surgery, and aftercare from surgeon and audiologist must also be considered. In the UK the operation and device is covered by the NHS but will cost approximately £8000 for surgery and device if done in a private hospital.

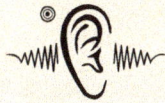

To Baha® or
to not Baha®

After great deliberation I decided to take up the offer of the Baha®. By this time I had been living with single-sided deafness for seven years and whilst I had got used to placing myself in situations where my lack of hearing wouldn't be too much of a hindrance to me there was still lots of times when I had trouble joining in conversations due to interference from background noise.

I soon received the appointment to have the abutment implant. It was to be in April 2011 just a few months after the initial chance meeting with the chap from Audiology.

It was strange to be back in a hospital bed after all those years (although as my baby son had been born in the same hospital just two months previously I was by no means a stranger to the place).

The Baha® abutment installation isn't a long operation and I was only to be on the ward for a day. I arrived early in the morning, and was given the usual induction to hospital life.

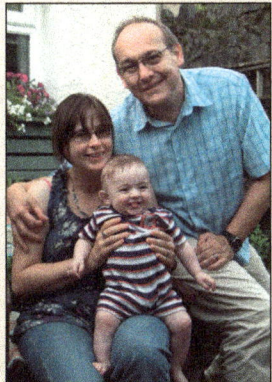

Photo by Ania Yoncali

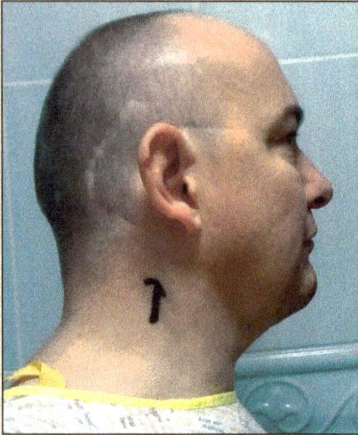

I decided to get my hair cut very short for the operation. The scar from the AN operation has totally healed but is still clearly visible.

I had an arrow drawn on my neck to remind the surgeon which side to operate on. The implantation of the Baha® is a simple procedure done in the operating room which takes approximately 1 hour. I was given the choice of general or local anaesthetic ... I chose general! A special skin graft is performed behind the deaf ear, and the skin follicles and fat are removed from the scalp.

Mmmmmm toast

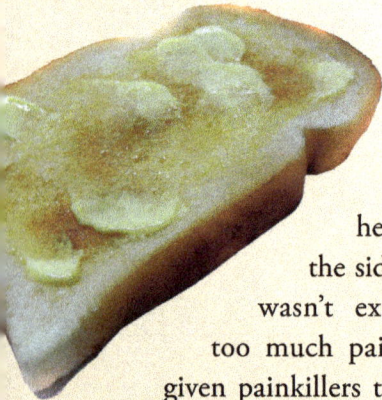

I soon awoke from the anaesthetic and I was famished – the nurse came and fluffed my pillows then brought me the best piece of toast I have ever eaten.

I have a bandage covering my head which soon slips off. The nerves at the side of head never regained feeling so I wasn't experiencing too much pain – I was given painkillers though and an appointment to visit the nurse in a few days time.

As you can see from the images the bandage was quite bloody, and

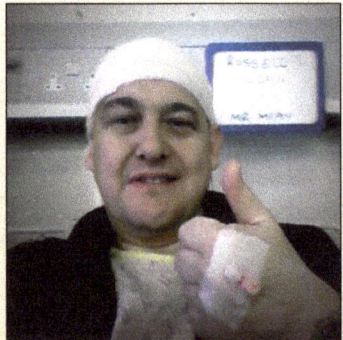

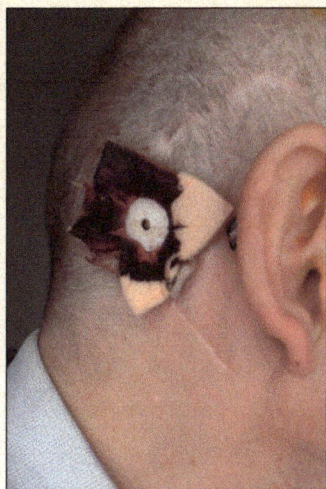

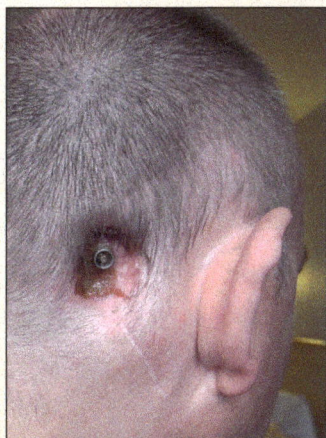

this had to remain in place for a few days which meant I had to go out in public with it, including work! I couldn't even wear a hat to cover it so I felt sorry for anyone stuck behind me who suddenly came across the sight of a post-op, blood soaked bandage. Just note the white disc on the left hand image – this was used to clip onto the abutment and hold the dressing in place... we'll come back to this handy little object later in the book.

I visited the ENT nurse a couple of days later – a nice lady called Marie – who was used to dealing with abutments. She gave me some advice about the care and main-tenance of it and recommended cleaning it daily. I was given a brush that resembles a toothbrush but with very very soft bristles. I was to use to clean the area with the brush and was also given small tube of Bactroban®, an anti-bacterial cream for tender areas! This was to prove a great asset over the following years.

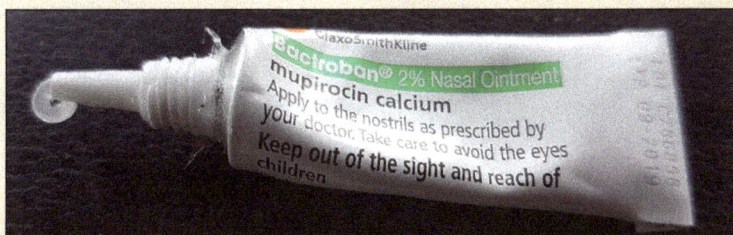

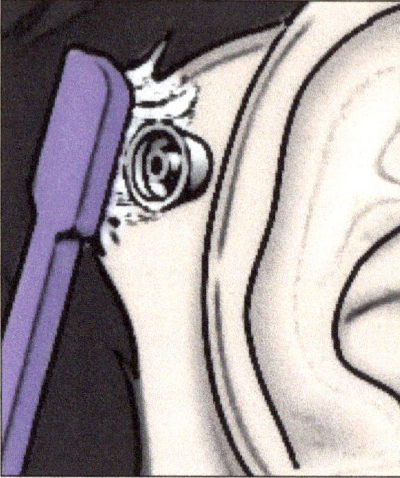

To be honest, the brush seemed to be quite useless – the abutment has a tendency to collect dead skin cells that produce a ring of scab! To clean off something as crusty as a scab with a soft bristled brush is like trying to clean day-old porridge off a cereal bowl with a tissue! I wash my hair every day so kept it clean.

An alternative method is to use a babywipe or similar to wipe around the area in a flossing manner. Easy? hmmm remember this is behind the ear, it's easier to lick your elbow!

The area soon healed, I had weekly, then fortnightly visits to the nurse for a month or so then was given the all-clear.

This was in April – it would be a further 3 months before I could return for the Hearing Aid.

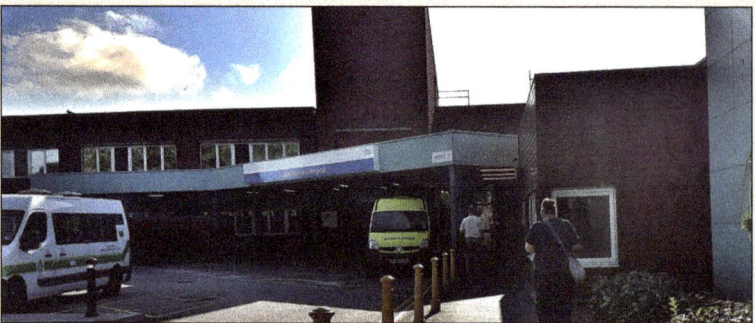

Audiology at furness General Hospital in Barrow-in-Furness

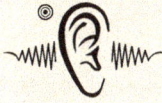

Living with a Baha®

The three months wait soon passed, and so in July 2011 the appointment for the 'hand-over' of the Baha® arrived.

To set it up correctly the audiologist plugged it into the PC first and programmed the device to acceptable volume levels for my hearing needs.

The hearing aid was then clipped snugly in place on the press stud fastener on the abutment. After a bit of tweaking, I was good to go. I immediately noticed the difference, sounds were amplified and more defined - It was a strange sensation covering my 'good' ear and still being to hear noises in the room.

I walked out with a spring in my step and stereo (ish) hearing for the first time in seven years!

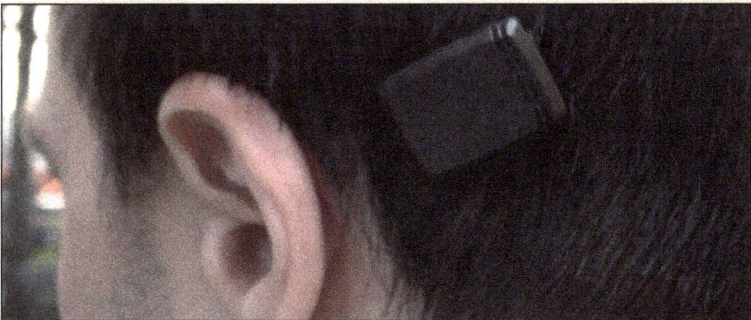

Someone else's head borrowed for illustrative purposes

Unboxing the Baha

The Baha is supplied with a good collection of accessories and instruction books.

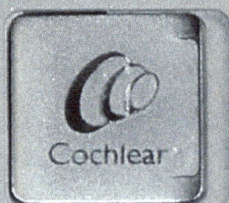

A large box with foam insert for the Baha & all accessories. (Subsequent models came in a less impressive cardboard bo

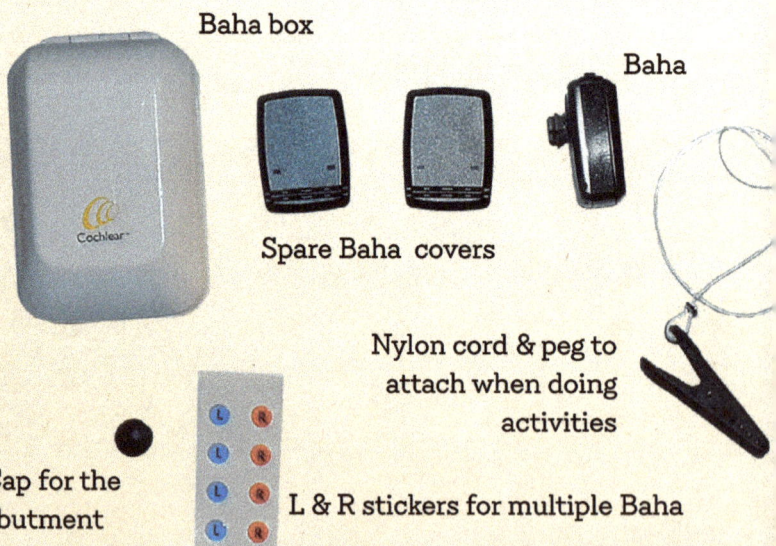

Baha box

Baha

Spare Baha covers

Nylon cord & peg to attach when doing activities

Cap for the abutment

L & R stickers for multiple Baha

Plastic post that fits the Baha to allow others to experience the way it conducts sound.

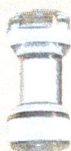

Soft bristle brush for cleaning the abutment area

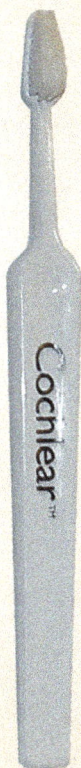

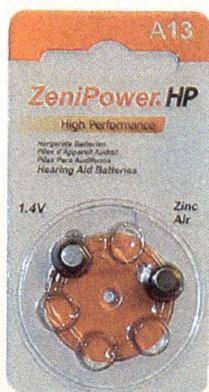

A13

ZeniPower. HP
High Performance

Norgerate Batteries
Piles d'Appareil Auditif
Pilas Para Audifonos
Hearing Aid Batteries

1.4V   Zinc
              Air

Cochlear™

Hearing aid batteries

Handy magnetic 'wand' to assist in the removal of batteries.

A Baha® takes a bit of getting used to. At first, there is a lot of fumbling as you tentatively try to clip the device into the orifice on the side of your head which you can't see even looking in a mirror. If you miss and try to put it between the abutment and the skin, it's very tender. But then you hear a reassuring 'click', and it's in place.

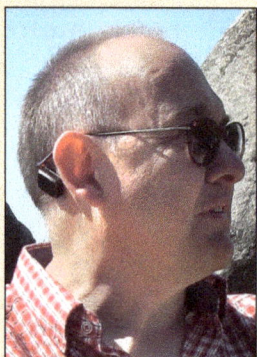

In situ it feels very firm, when you tap in with your finger, it feels well fixed in place although it can spin freely on its fixing. This fumbling occurs for a few days, but then with regular use, it becomes second nature, and at times you even forget you are wearing it ... like wearing spectacles – you know you have got used to them when you accidentally leave them on when you go to bed.

On the subject of Glasses, I find that whenever I get a new pair, I have to chop a couple of centimetres off the right arm, or else it has a tendency to touch the Baha® and causes feedback.

You have to remember it is there, though, as you are sporting an expensive piece of technical equipment clipped to your head. The press stud is very good, although I have experienced the

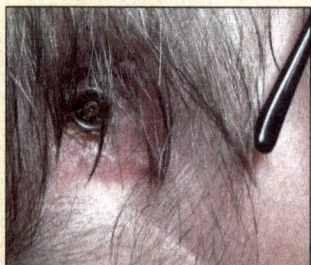

Baha® pop out on a few occasions - usually when you find yourself changing a tyre, or helping a neighbour move their piano. You have to remember to remove it when taking a shower, doing any sports activity and definitely when going for a swim! The Baha® unit is supplied

with a clip attached to thin nylon cord that can be looped around the unit and used when engaging in physical activities to prevent it getting lost if it pops out in all the excitement!

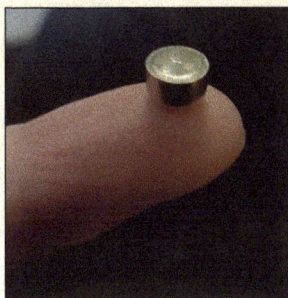

The Baha® is powered by a typical button cell 'hearing aid' battery which is simple although slightly fiddly to change (but which hearing aids don't have fiddly batteries?)... You'd think for a gizmo that is used primarily for the older end of the population who tend to suffer more with bad eyesight and shaky hands that there would be a better way of powering hearing aids ... everything is rechargeable in this day and age, why not hearing aids?

As well as the improved amplification from the hearing aid there are also a lot of unwanted noises that are amplified too. Feedback is a familiar sound for any hearing aid user - the loud whistle-screech noise that suddenly cries like a banshee, or the noise of the wind cracking through the device like the devil's cough. I always said that if they ever invented a fluffy cover like the ones you see on an outdoor microphone for the Baha I'd be first in the queue! The noise made by the device when it isn't connected to the abutment is also very unnerving. It of course vibrates and occasionally has 'woken up' in the night on my night-stand and sounds like a giant bee doing a tap dance!

Over the next few weeks though all was not plain sailing – I got a lot more feedback that normal from the device, especially when it was turned up even slightly. I found I couldn't use it except in almost quiet circumstances. I would bring this up at my next appointment.

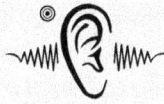

Magnets & Metal Detectors

Sometimes it's easy to forget there is a titanium screw implanted into the skull as a permanent fixture. Because of this, in the box of accessories that comes with the Baha is a set of credit card sized information sheets. There are two types of card printed in several languages.

One of them is to take along on vacation, to show the security staff at airports if the metal detectors suddenly start buzzing as you walk past them. The card explains the implant and its purpose. I have been through a couple of airports since the implant, including a trip to the USA where the metal detectors are set to maximum without any issues... but always take the cards to be on the safe side.

The other card is to show medical staff if ever a trip to an MRI scan is required. An encounter with a giant magnet is probably not the best thing you go into without first mentioning you have a metal screw in the skull. It is OK to have an MRI scan with a BAHA. All patients undergoing MRI scans are asked whether they have any metallic implants. Strong magnetic fields inside the scanner could cause ferrous metal to move, and this could injure the patient. But the BAHA fixture and abutment are made of titanium. Titanium is non-magnetic. You will still need to take off the sound processor to go into the scanner.

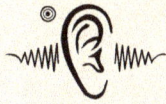

Adventures in re-fashioning part 1

It turned out that the skin around the abutment was protruding and touching the hearing aid – as a result, it wasn't able to do its job efficiently and was producing feedback. The conclusion was that I had to have another operation on the site to 're-fashion' the skin.

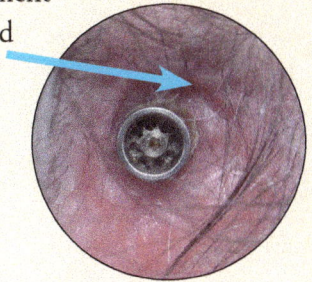

So in October 2011 (just six months after the original surgery) I found myself in the hospital again. The visit was similar to the last time, and before long I was wearing the Baha® again.

After the re-fashioning, the feedback was reduced, and the audiologist was able to increase the volume limit – but it wasn't perfect, I still got feedback and really didn't use it that often, only in situations where I expected big crowds.

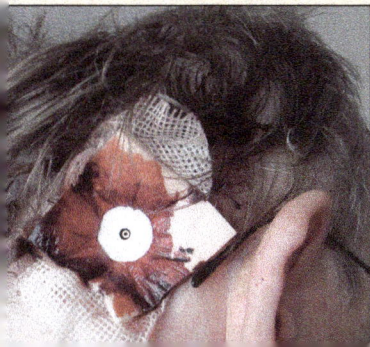

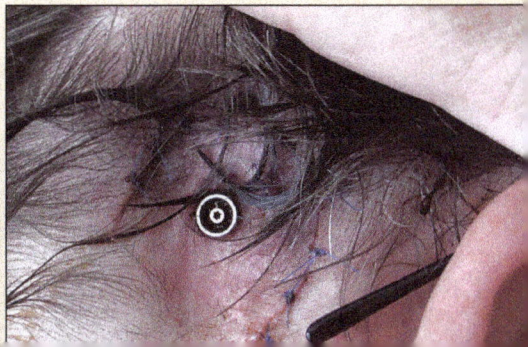

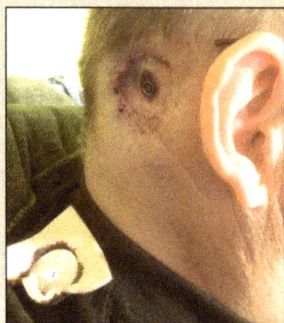

This routine continued for the next 12 months or so.

I also experienced quite a bit of infection on the abutment site; it would often get sore, and sometimes bleed. This soreness was exacerbated at night with rubbing on my pillow – I remembered the plastic disc that held my dressing on which I had put away in a drawer. (The disc, not the bloody dressing that is). The disc – about the size of a 1p coin clipped onto the abutment and acted as a protective cover for the site around the abutment. It worked – whenever the site was infected or sore I'd use the cover for a few nights and it would soon heal up – it's been the most useful bit of kit I have owned over the past few years! I even once asked at the hospital about buying a spare in case it got lost, the company that supplies them charges £30 for the disc!

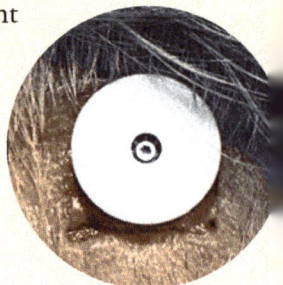

I also used the Bactroban® cream to good effect. My hair is always short but I'd notice when it got to a particular length it would irritate the abutment site for a week or so and would often get infected.

So this was the routine for the next couple of years – the Baha® would be worn most of the time but only turned on when needed and at night the plastic disc would be worn to prevent friction.

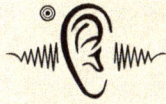

Adventures in re-fashioning part 2

In Spring 2014 I experienced quite a prolonged period of infection. One evening I went to clip the disc in place and found it was quite painful to do so. The next day I couldn't wear my Baha®, and the next night I couldn't get the disc on at all - the skin had grown over half of the abutment.

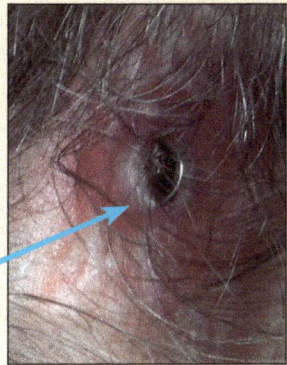

The case of the disappearing abutment

I made an appointment to see the nurse a few days later, and she confirmed the skin had 'invaded' the abutment. I had to see the consultant who told me I'd have to have more surgery to re-re-fashion the area.

It was to be almost six months before I got the appointment to return to the hospital. In that time the Baha® returned

to its box, and I went through months without using any hearing device. As time went on I found I didn't miss it as much as I thought, and by the time I got the appointment I was even having second thoughts about having the operation.

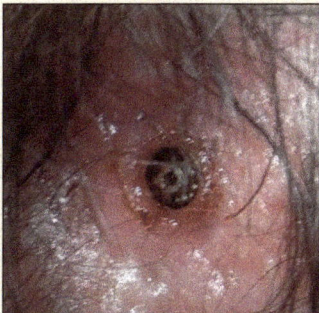

By now the skin had grown over most of the abutment, and I wondered whether the hassle of having the Baha® was worth it. The infections, the nightly use of the disc, the constant cleaning, the regular trips to the operating theatre, etc seems a lot to cope with compared to the practical use of the Baha® on a daily basis.

I wanted to speak to the consultant before the operation but unfortunately despite three appointments he was either on holiday, sick or behind schedule so it had to be cancelled. It wasn't until the actual day of the operation that I got to see him when he visited me for a pre-op check. I had lots of questions, but there was now no time to discuss them – it came down to a yes or no.

I decided to stick with the Baha®. I had the operation; the site was re-re-fashioned, and a steroid injection was put in the area to prevent the skin growing over the site again.

The result of this re-re-fashioning is a further extension to the ugly scar I have on my head. I have very little hair to hide it and get quite self-conscious about it. I mostly wear the Baha® to hide this scarred area than actually as a hearing aid.

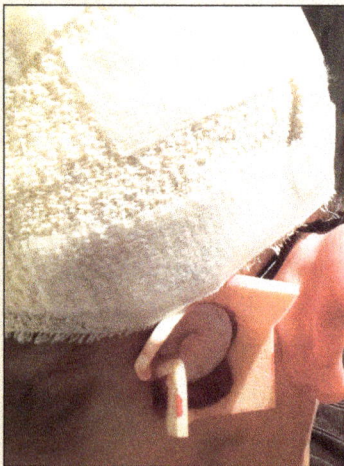

In January 2015, because I'd had the Baha® for three years I was given an update to the latest model, the Cochlear™ Baha® 4. The Baha® 4 looks physically the same as the previous model but has had a serious hardware upgrade and now uses wireless technology. I must admit the sound quality is much improved and along with the recent re-re-fashioning I hardly experience feedback these days.

Along with the upgraded hearing aid I was given another exciting piece of equipment – a wireless mini-microphone. The Mini Microphone is a portable wireless clip-on microphone that transmits speech and sound directly to the sound processor. It clips onto the collar of a companion, and in a noisy environment like a restaurant or sporting event (or even shopping with the missus) it enables me to hear them speak clearly and directly through the sound processor. The hype is better than actual usage – there are cut outs, the range isn't brilliant and connecting is a bit of a faff. Still it's better than nothing!

The newest version of the Baha®, the Baha® 5, has been unveiled at the time of writing – with even better technology with its own remote control smart phone app - I look forward to my next upgrade in 2017!

Along with the recent updates to the system there is now also a new method of attaching the Baha®. The abutment, which is now magnetic, is fitted under the skin so is less conspicuous. Known as the 'attract' method as opposed to the current 'connect' method. Great news! Unfortunately, this is too late for me ... it would certainly have ensured no nasty scars!

Fingers crossed there'll be no need for re-re-re-fashioning!

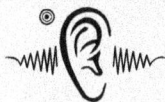

Abutment news

In November 2016, guess what? The problem re-occurred. I experienced the same issue as in spring 2014 – the skin invaded the abutment area almost overnight. I got an appointment for ENT who examined the latest skinning over of the abutment. I was given anti-biotics to take down the swelling and told a further meeting would be made with the consultant.

In March 2017 I finally got to see the consultant, he had a look and confirmed the problem had occurred yet again, and so I asked the big question - "should it stay or should it go?" My main concern is that if it is removed, I'd be at a disadvantage further down the line if I experienced deafness in my 'good' ear in years to come. Was a removal reversible? The answer was yes it was. Even if the abutment is removed the fixing screw in the skull remains in place (as this is now knitted to the bone anyway). There was a slightly 'crossed wire' at the meeting however when he thought I was requesting the abutment be removed there and then. He popped out of the room and returned 2 minutes later with Michelle from the Audiology department. She was armed with a mini torque wrench set aimed at my head. I quickly explained I had just been considering options and didn't want it removing that very day! The audiologist had a look and confirmed that it was too skinned over to have removed it in the clinic even if I had wanted to.

We had a good chat, and she mentioned it may be a good idea to try a longer abutment before I give up on the whole Baha® idea. We had to first get the skin invasion sorted out, so the forms were filled out for an operation to remove the skin and replace the short abutment with a longer one.

Amazingly, during the summer months of 2017, the skin abated itself. The abutment cleared, and I was able to use my hearing aid once again. I had a routine appointment booked at Audiology in July, and it was still completely clear by then.

The main reason for my visit to Audiology was to meet up with the Cochlear™ rep. It was to discuss the longer abutment and the feasibility of replacing my Baha for the new magnetic connect system that Cochlear™ have developed. It was great to talk to him about the process, the hearing aids and the company itself.

The Cochlear™ Baha® Connect System is a well-proven bone conduction hearing system featuring the minimally invasive DermaLock™ technology. This technology helps preserve the hair and skin around the abutment. Alas, I had missed the boat for the Baha® Connect System. It seems now that the abutment connector for new Bahas has a different connector to the one I had fitted 6 years ago. To take advantage of the new magnetic Baha® Connect System version, I would have to have a second implant, positioned in a different place in my skull (around 4 cm higher than it is now). This would then be fitted with the new type of abutment. Obviously, the downside to this would be that I'd still have a significant scarred area with an obsolete screw and another abutment further up.

They arranged another appointment and gave me the use of an Alice band to test the Connect style of hearing aid for a few weeks. To also consider the alternative of having a longer abutment installed.

After some consideration, I decided that my best option was to stick with the existing fixing and to have a longer abutment installed instead. The magnetic Baha® Connect System is excellent, and it would have been ideal to have the option from the beginning, but obviously, it wasn't available then.

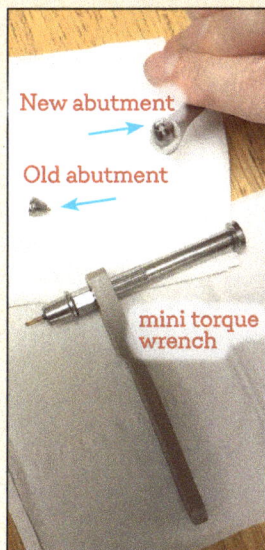

New abutment

Old abutment

mini torque wrench

Because the area was still clear of extra skin, I could have the abutment replaced in the clinic without the need for an operation. The time had come for Michelle the Audiologist to get her mini torque wrench out again. The sensation of having a bolt screwed out of one's skull is one I won't forget - it didn't hurt at all - it was just a strange sensation. The new bolt being screwed in felt even stranger still. The result was a brand new abutment that protrudes about 3mm above the skin rather than on the surface as before. The Baha® sits on there without touching the skin as before although it is more prone to getting knocked off at times.

The good news is that I haven't had to wear the plastic disc over it at night since

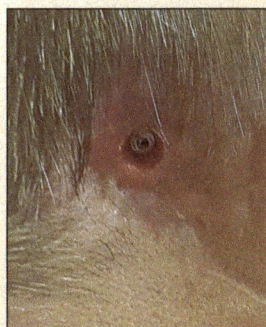

Midway between the old & the new, the lower screw can be seen clearly.

having it fitted. Fast forward 3 months - it's now November 2017 and I have just taken possession of a brand new Baha® 5.

The Baha® 5 is a major update by Cochlear™. It has had a major upgrade in its technology and is smaller than its predecessors. They say good things come in small packages.

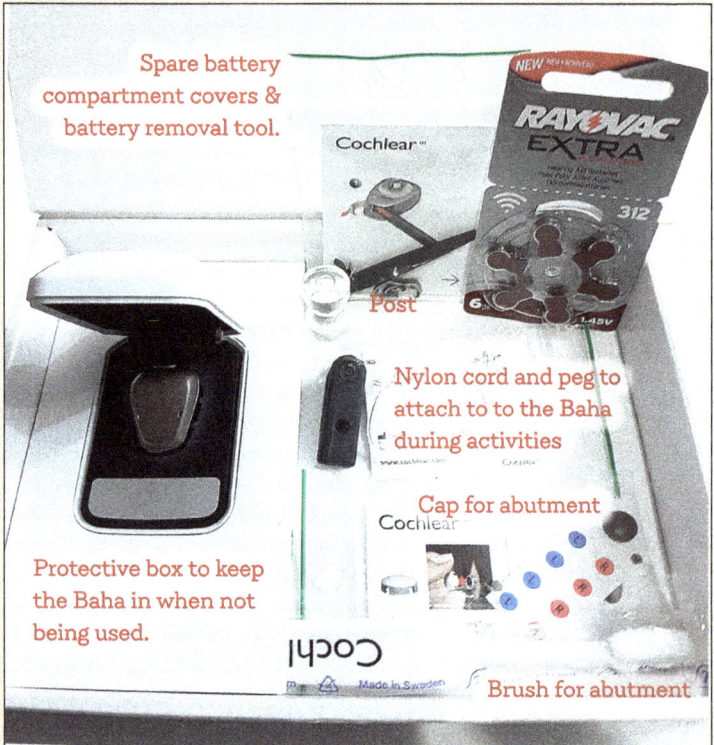

The Baha® 5 Sound Processor looks like a beetle and has been specially re-designed to let the wearer enjoy their listening experience and better hearing, even in noisy environments. An all-new smart chip drives the latest, most advanced automatic technologies that constantly monitor surroundings.

The sound processor makes seamless adjustments to enhance and focus on the important things the wearer needs to hear.

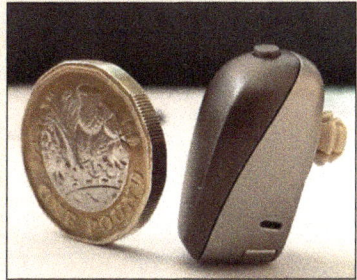

So far, I'm pleased with the clearer sound quality and bluetooth capabilities of the new hearing aid. The volume is set at fitting and the **only way** to manually adjust is via a phone app the **Baha 5 Smart**. In theory the app connects your phone to the hearing aid so that the volume can be controlled remotely. This was great until a recent upgrade to a newer phone then it stopped working. It turns out that Cochlear™ don't keep their apps updated on a regular basis thus making features of their newest hearing aids defunct.

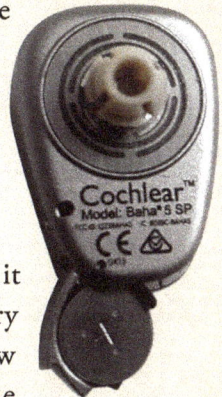

Strangely the only way to turn it off though is to open the battery cover. This is an obvious design flaw as they now also supply extra battery compartments in the box as the catch is prone to wearing out quickly.

Unfortunately the unit is still not rechargeable.

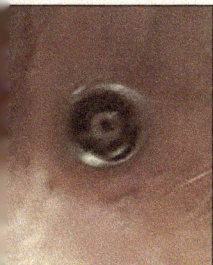

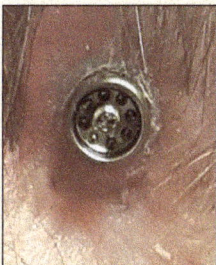

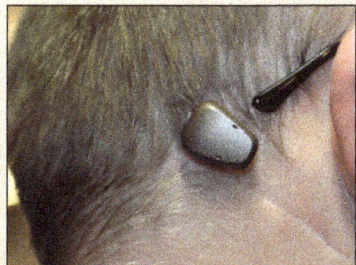

The 'old' abutment

The new longer abutment

Wearing the Baha 5

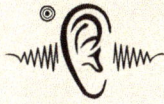

And Finally...

Even though the operation to remove the Acoustic Neuroma was so long ago its legacy still hangs over me. It's been interesting to read back the diary entries and realise the things that are normal to me today were brand new feelings and experiences back then. I've totally forgotten what it was like to hear in stereo, and single-sided deafness is just a part of who I am.

Profile of my life now

HEARING - My right side hearing will of course never return, but as the years have gone by, I have got used to it. I still pick my spot to maximise amplification. Due to the nature of my business, I often attend networking events. In essence, I find these very difficult, even with my hearing aid set to warp factor ten. I find myself still nodding at conversations I only half hear and hold back from asking too much in case they've already told me the thing I want to ask! I was recently excluded from a business trip to a trade show in an exhibition hall because I was told my deafness would mean I couldn't communicate well with others in a noisy environment. This was the first time in the 14 years of being deaf I have experienced such an exclusion because of this disability and is a stark reminder that I'm not as effective as I once was and have to remember my limitations.

105

Having the Bone Anchored Hearing Aid has of course changed my hearing experience. It adds a new dimension to my hearing ability and has added a surround sound capability. On the other hand I'm now more conscious of my deafness. Up until the fitting I was inconspicuous in my deafness, there was no visible sign I was deaf in the right ear, whilst now there is a big arrow in the shape of a clip-on hearing aid.

BALANCE - Although in the main, this has not been a problem for me as time has progressed, I still find it disconcerting to walk around in the dark.

There are times I feel clumsy, it's a similar feeling to the way you have to concentrate on each step when walking across stepping stones in a river – or after you have had one too many glasses of wine and you try to walk as if you are perfectly sober ... I have had several ferry journeys in the past few years and found this phenomenon magnified. However, on the plus side, I didn't feel seasick!

I still feel uncomfortable with my back towards the room - because there is no hearing or balance on the right side it makes me feel uneasy, the same kind of feeling as when you are blindfolded and don't know where everyone is and have that expectation that someone is suddenly going to grab you. I can still ride a bike with no problem as long as I don't look over my shoulder while I'm doing it.

FACIAL PARALYSIS - My face has never returned to its pre-op flexibility. In a state of relaxation my face looks 'normal' but when I make big facial gestures one half always looks happier than the other. My eye now closes properly but still gets crusty when I am tired or when it's windy ... generally it's not a problem though.

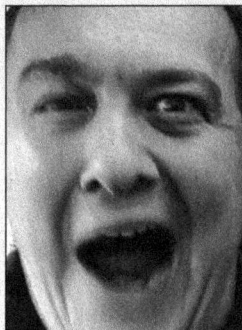

IN GENERAL - I still find I get 'suddenly tired'. It's as if I get to a certain point then switch off rather than a progressive winding down.

I still have tinnitus. At times worse than others but I have again grown accustomed to it. It's the 'washing machine' type these days - although it's as if the washing machine is in another room not right there with me. (if that makes sense).

My memory is not what it used to be - before the operation I used to pride myself in remembering people's names and people would often comment on it. Now I struggle to call my four children by their correct names! I often need to give myself a skill refresher when returning to a process that I have not done for just a few weeks - even if I had regularly done the same process for months beforehand. I find taking notes helps. I seem to go through phases where I am 'bright as a button' then suddenly struggle to remember what day it is almost.

MENTAL HEALTH - During the past few years I have divorced, remarried, moved house three times, been made redundant and started a new business, had three lots of Baha® surgery, had two more children and have become a grandad.

Although, I suppose whether I'd had the acoustic neuroma operation or not these things would still have over-faced me. I do go through more bouts of depression since 2004 than previously, and I have to fight a 'can't do' attitude that prevents me from doing things on occasion. But I quickly got up fighting again.

In 2012, after working at the educational publishers for over seven years, I started my own business, Pixel Tweaks, offering Graphic Design services.

During the years since then, I have specialised in book production and publishing services for self-publishers. I have helped over sixty authors get more than 100 books in print and published. Over the years several of these books have been shortlisted in the Lakeland Book of

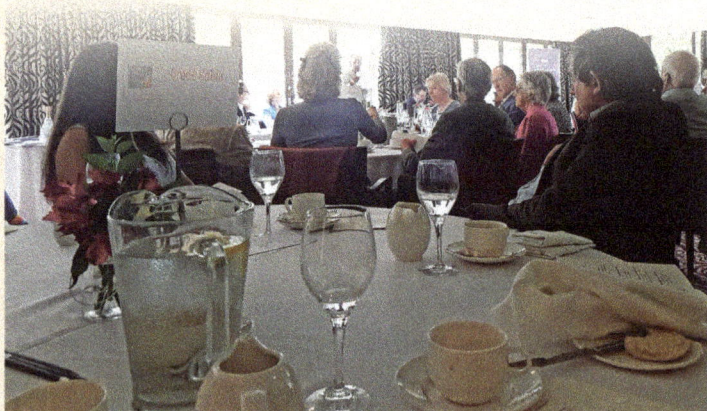

2017 Lakeland Book of the Year Award

the Year Awards which is always a great accolade for all involved.

Providing this service for others was what encouraged me to put my own experiences together from the information that I had accumulated about Acoustic Neuroma and Baha since 2004 into book form too. I entered a copy of this book in the 2017 Lakeland Book of the Year Award. Though it wasn't shortlisted, it was long-listed and given a special mention by the esteemed author Hunter Davies which I was delighted about.

Is this the end of the story? I've come to the conclusion that following an acoustic neuroma operation, there is no 'end' of the story ... well, there will be 'AN' end, but that's the last thing that will happen! (see addendum).

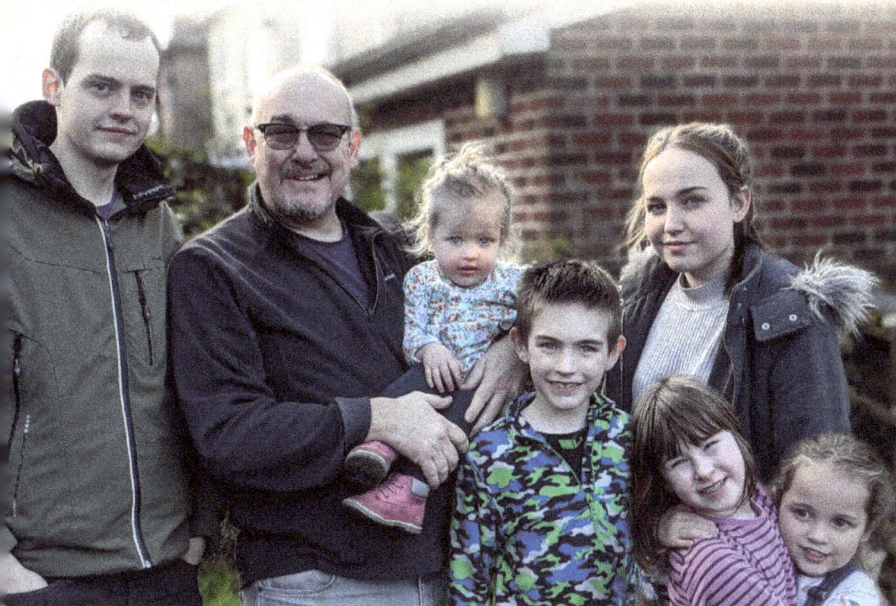

February 2020 with my four beautiful children and two Granddaughters.

Acoustic Nemesis

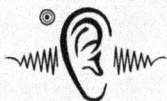

Addendum

(or should that be abutment?)

In 2020 after much deliberation, I decided to part ways with my BAHA system. For too long the peg has been a source of constant irritation. As mentioned already in the book, this is an open wound that refuses to heal properly. At night it rubs on the pillow causing more irritation leading to soreness and bleeding and infection then more irritation. This cycle has beleaguered me for the past nine years. I can hold my hand up and say I've given it a good shot, I've put up with several re-fashionings and changes of pegs, so I'm going to finally concede that this is not the best solution for me.

If the Cochlear hearing aid worked well and was making a real difference in my life, I would be persuaded to put up with this discomfort, but since Baha 5 the system hasn't been as efficient as previous versions. Cochlear did away with volume controls on the Baha 5, and instead, they created a smart-phone app (primarily for iPhones) to control the volume remotely. However, they have failed to keep the app updated. The app did work for Android phones up until 2017 then stopped. On the Android app store, it currently has a very low rating with many people complaining at the lack of updates for Android users and leaving negative reviews about the app. Unfortunately, it suggests perhaps Cochlear isn't making app development a priority at the moment; hence, the hearing aid remains unfit for purpose for many users.

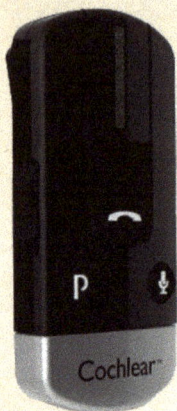

Image Courtesy of Cochlear™

There is a work-around. I was given a second piece of equipment to use which acts as a volume control for the Baha, but with the best will in the world, it means remembering to bring that gizmo with you which means carrying something the size of a car key remote around. Plus it has to be turned on and paired with the hearing aid to work which again is another process to worry about.

So in early March 2020, I visited Audiology to have the abutment removed. It was done by the Cochlear rep who had the 'right tool for the job' (see p101). The job took just a few seconds and was painless. The abutment had to go off to 'the lab' to check it for nasties - pity, it would have been a good keepsake!

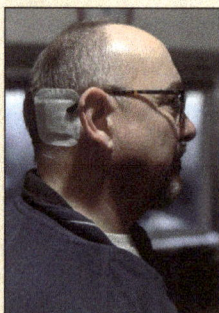

I had to return to the hospital a week later as the lab had found traces of Streptococcus, so I was given a course of antibiotics.

The Cochlear rep suggested a couple of alternatives I might like to try including the Cochlear BAHA SoundArc - a headband setup with the BAHA attached. It seems like an excellent non-surgical, non-invasive alternative that can be slipped on and off according to the situation... so, watch this space.

The week after these appointments we went into lockdown with the Covid-19 pandemic, so everything was put on hold anyway.

The hole left by the removed abutment has healed well, there is a slight indent where it used to be but nothing too noticeable as you can see in this photo.

So here ends my saga. Hopefully, now the abutment has gone my acoustic nemesis will keep quiet, and I'll have nothing else to write about on the subject.

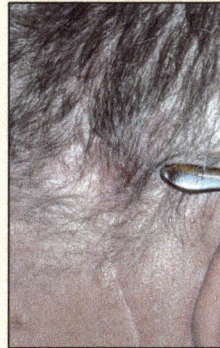

Thanks for listening to my rambling and I hope it has given anyone facing the challenges of Acoustic Neuroma surgery some encouragement and positivity for the future.

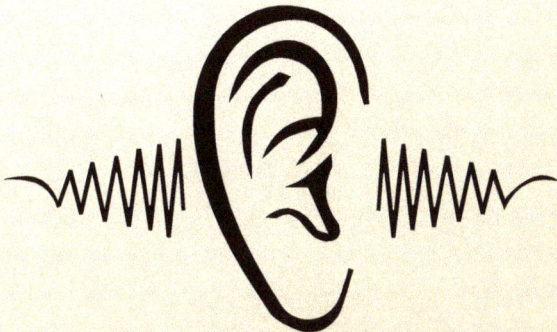

Index

Acoustic Nemesis

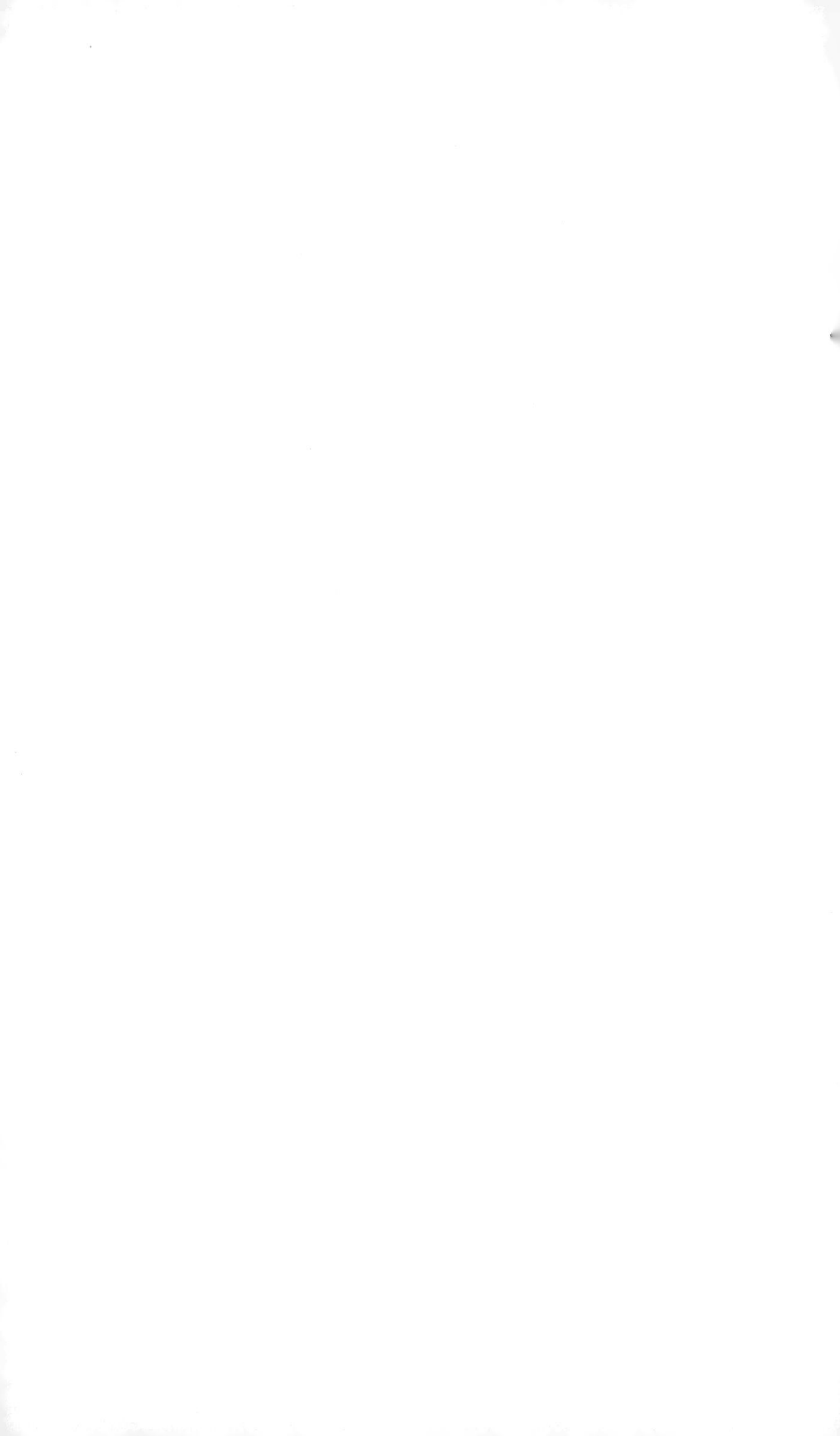

www.ingramcontent.com/pod-product-compliance
Lightning Source LLC
Chambersburg PA
CBHW051246020426
42333CB00025B/3086